Love in the time of Medical School:

Build a happy, healthy relationship with a medical student

Printed in the United States of America

Cover by Andy Highland

ISBN-13: 978-1546625988

ISBN-10: 1546625984

Philadelphia, PA, 19107

www.DatingMed.com

For Brian

My everything.

TABLE OF CONTENTS

CHAPTER 1
INTRODUCTION

"No story is a straight line. The geometry of a human life is too imperfect and complex, too distorted by the laughter of time and the bewildering intricacies of fate to admit the straight line into its system of laws."
— Pat Conroy, *Beach Music*

I remember sitting on the couch in our Miami apartment, looking out the window and thinking, *there is so much I wish I had known.* It was 2014, and my fiancé Brian was three years into medical school and I was between jobs. Despite the beautiful palm trees, I struggled to feel at home in Miami — a city I moved to in 2013 to live near Brian while he completed his medical training. The decision to move was itself fraught with identity questions and self-doubt. (Examples of said questions include: Am I the kind of person who moves to a brand-new city for my boyfriend? What does that mean about me? Will that change the way people view me? Does this mean I value his career over mine?) Despite the exhausting internal dialogue, I made the plunge and moved to Florida. Now, while Brian and I planned our wedding and a future together, I began jotting down a list on the many unexpected challenges of dating a medical student, and how we addressed each one. I thought about our lack of time together... competitive stress... household responsibilities... the list kept growing. I started interviewing other med student significant others (SOs) about their experiences, a process that taught me so much about tough choices and made me feel less alone. I scoured Amazon for relevant books and the internet for articles about medical school and relationships. Armed with data, stories, and my own experiences, I began to write. What began as a five-page e-book turned into a much longer book. I need a nap.

Being the third wheel in a two-person relationship

From the time they start their first year, medical students enter into a long-term relationship with medicine. They have committed to a non-negotiable, closely held dream to which they have already pledged their time, energy, and money. Some would say that this relationship is monogamous, leaving little room for a human relationship. On many occasions, you will wonder how you became the third wheel in a two-person relationship. Still, we continue on and in the process, we experience what it is to be proud and lonely, excited and overwhelmed. We learn to traverse the landscape of American medicine, an opaque subculture with its own norms, language, and certainly, demands.

We are not alone in the struggle to adapt to our partner's career lifestyle. Lawyers, investment bankers, business owners, service workers, and many others work long and hard. Those dating consultants, techies, retail managers, and marketers also face the challenge of learning field-specific jargon. Medical students hold no monopoly on strange schedules or student debt. But still. Knowing that other fields require long hours does not make enduring medical school's hours any easier. Knowing that others are in debt does not ease the burden of addressing the financial realities of medical training. Other people's suffering does not make your own more tolerable — at best it provides empathic allies and perspective.

I started dating Brian when he was studying for the Medical College Admission Test (MCAT), a study period so intense that it may as well come with a giant banner reading "THIS IS JUST THE BEGINNING. RUNNNN!" Yet I didn't run. After we graduated from Brandeis University, Brian started medical school in Miami and I moved to Thailand for a year to teach English and travel around Southeast Asia. After returning from a year of independent living and travel, I made the decision to settle in Miami to try to build a life near Brian. I had no connections in the Miami area, not even a Great Aunt Esther to visit in Boca Raton. I anticipated the stressors of transition and the stressors of dating a graduate student. I did not anticipate the alternate reality of medical school. And throughout, it felt like Brian's needs came first — his schooling became *our* top priority. I struggled to be supportive and independent, building my own life in tandem with his. Things worked out for us; we got married during his fourth year of med school, and we are more in love than ever. But that outcome came from learning to cope with long stretches apart, negotiating household responsibilities, and prioritizing one another when it was easier not to.

If you are dating, engaged to, or married to a medical student, this book is for you. I will walk you through the mechanics and structure of medical school and teach you how to cope with the different sources of stress you may encounter.

There are several circumstances that I do not cover in this book: I do not directly address dual medical student relationships, which present unique challenges. I shied away from tackling the topic of raising children during medical school, and I do not speak extensively about the specifics of joint-degree programs (such as an MD/PHD), or international, military, osteopathic and podiatric program requirements. Still, I tried to be thorough.

Now, let's start at the beginning...

CHAPTER 2
THE APPLICATION PROCESS

"And this I believe: that the free, exploring mind of the individual human
is the most valuable thing in the world."
— John Steinbeck, East of Eden

If you start dating somebody who is applying to medical school, you will find yourself part of a time-consuming, stressful, expensive, and scary process that may raise some important questions about your relationship. But first, the application process itself need not be confusing. It is a multi-step process that operates on a specific timetable.

Part 1: In June, medical schools begin accepting the first part of the application called the primary applications, through AMCAS, the American Medical College Application Service. (Some Texas schools use the TDMSAS, the Texas Medical and Dental Schools Application Service, for their primary application because Texans like to do everything differently. As a Texan myself, I take great pride in our stubborn insensitivity to the plight of stressed-out, poor applicants.) A primary application consists of:

1. MCAT scores
2. The student's college transcripts and GPA
3. Letters of recommendation
4. Personal statement
5. Extracurricular activities list
6. An application fee (of course)

Part 2: Each medical school screens the primary applications, and applicants who pass muster receive their secondary application. Secondary applications vary but typically consist of:

1. More personal information
2. Additional essay questions, usually tailored to the specific school
3. Another application fee (of course)

Part 3: Medical schools review secondary applications and invite selected students to interview throughout the fall and winter. *Note: Students are expected to pay travel and lodging expenses.*

Part 4: Medical schools evaluate the students they interviewed. Students wait (im)patiently to hear back.

Part 5: Medical schools send out decisions. Students may initially be placed on a wait list, with the final decision coming later.

Do I get a say?

Medical school applications can raise big hairy questions about the long-term potential and trajectory of your relationship.

- Does our relationship factor into where they apply?
- Do I get a say in where they choose to go to school?
- Is our relationship going to stay intact?
- What if we're not on the same page?
- How do we even talk about this stuff?

For some, these questions arise in synchrony with your relationship — at a time when you and your partner are thinking about your long-term prospects. But for those in newer relationships, these questions feel out of place. Unfortunately for medical couples, this will be only one of many times when medical training forces you to address relationship questions on its own schedule.

If your relationship is not yet serious, it may feel as though it is too soon to have a say in your partner's decision. When Brian applied to school, we had been dating for a little over a year, and while I supported him through the process, I stayed out of the decision-making because we did not yet know whether our relationship would endure. When he received his acceptances, we discussed the options together and talked about what would be in his best interest.

If you are married, engaged, or otherwise committed to a long-term relationship, application decisions may feel like a joint task. Those conversations (and there will be many) may include discussing each of your priorities, including what schools and locations best meet both of your needs. How committed partners make these decisions differs based on the couple. Some non-applicants want a say in where the student applies. Others only want a say in the final decision once acceptances arrive. Still others feel untethered to geography and will gladly live wherever the student needs to go. Ultimately, how the two of you negotiate this will be based on the seriousness of your relationship and your needs.

The ability to discuss these overarching questions will prove a fundamental skill throughout your partner's medical training. It is normal for this process to be hard — these are huge questions. This might be the first time that the two of you conceptualize this life step as a joint venture — something you want to face together. If the two of you are struggling, it will help to understand what this process brings up for you or your partner. Here are some possible scenarios:

- My partner and I have never made a big joint decision before. The stakes feel high, and I'm afraid we'll make a bad decision and they'll resent me later.
- It seems like one of us feels more committed to our relationship than the other; one of us thinks it should be an individual decision and the other thinks it should be a joint decision.
- My partner does not share decision-making power well. They feel they should make this decision without my input, and I should simply agree to it. (This can be reversed)

- My partner seems really stressed out by the application process, and it makes it hard to understand how they feel about my involvement in the process.

Thinking about these options and others will help you address the real underlying fear in this already complicated process. Most of these are struggles that can be overcome through open communication and negotiation. One thing to be aware of is whether your partner otherwise shares power well. In married couples, inability to share power and influence is a red flag, and generally men are guiltier of this than women. Among married couples, if a man is unwilling to share power and influence, the marriage had an 81 percent chance of leading to divorce.[1] How do you figure out whether your partner feels uncomfortable with you having a say in this decision specifically versus this being a bigger trend where you feel shut out? Reflect on other big decisions — did you feel that the two of you approached the decision together? Can you think of other examples when you have felt excluded?

It may turn out that the two of you are not on the same page regarding how much influence you should wield in this decision. In this case, they may struggle to convey their thoughts without hurting your feelings. Here are some ways to approach the topic using "I statements" that do not have an accusatory tone:

- I am feeling left out of the application process. Can we talk about whether I have a role in this?
- I am feeling pushed away. How can I support you right now?
- This whole process is bringing up scary questions for me about our future. Is it doing the same for you?

How to support your partner

Even if the two of you decide that it is too soon for you to have a say in the process, you can still get involved — here are a few suggestions for how:

- Offer to listen while they vent about the process
- Help research potential schools and cities

1   John Mordechai Gottman and Nan Silver, *The seven principles for making marriage work: a practical guide from the country's foremost relationship expert* (New York: Harmony Books, 2015).

- If you are a writer or editor, offer to edit their personal statement
- Practice interviewing with them
- Help them blow off steam

At the beginning of application season, you might say something like, *"This process is going to be stressful, and I want to support you however I can. What can I do to help you? What do you need from me?"* Different applicants will want different levels and types of help, and the only way to know what you can do is to ask. If they respond by saying, "I do not know," list some of the ways you'd be willing to help. If they want to handle the process by themselves, offer to help them blow off steam when they get stressed out.

This decision may be the first time that you and your partner feel stress about medical school at the same time. What I mean is, the application process will be stressful for both of you — yes, you too! And you both have a right to feel stress about the application process. They will be worrying about getting into school, paying for school, moving for school, and getting started. You may be worried about moving for their schooling, adjusting to the new stressors, and navigating your role and how the outcome will impact your collective future. That is no small thing. Notice the times when the two of you feel stressed out about medical school at the same time. Try to notice if you start judging your own stress. It can be easy to think that because you are not the applicant, you are not entitled to feel stress about medical training. Guess what — you are. It will be different stress, but legitimate nonetheless.

Finishing with the medical school application cycle can feel like a relief, and certainly it is. But one significant other (SO) I interviewed put it this way: "As a girlfriend, you are like, 'Finally, he's in! He's accepted. Now we have a life.' But no; it is only the beginning."

Moving for your partner

As we have said, the road to becoming a doctor forces couples at each juncture to make relationship judgments and decisions that may feel out of sync with the seriousness of the relationship. A couple that has dated for only four months, for example, may face the reality of a medical school acceptance across the country and the question of whether one partner should move for another. That gesture and its implications can feel better suited to a couple that has dated for substantially longer. If you decide to move for your partner, there are a few things you can do to ease the transition.

Talk with your partner about how it feels to move for them. They may not realize that you are worried about the symbolism of the gesture. Decide together how you want to view and talk about the move. Control how you see the decision. Moving for your partner does not have to mean that your relationship is taking on a new level of seriousness. No — moving for your partner only signals that you are flexible and medical school's rigid requirements force you to exercise that flexibility. If moving feels too permanent, adding another level of stress to the decision, decide to think of the move as a reversible adventure. Moving feels permanent but it is not. It is a pain in the butt, but can change if the relationship doesn't work out. Decide that you are OK making the decision that's best for you at this moment.

The most important thing to do when you decide to move for a partner is to take responsibility for the decision. Own the choice and decide that you will not resent your partner if things does not work out. In fact, if you decide to move for your partner, say the following sentence out loud:

"I am going to [Insert City Name Here] because I made an adult decision. I accept the consequences if the city makes me unhappy or the relationship doesn't last. I'm an adult, and I'm owning this decision."

Your decision about whether to follow your significant other to medical school should not be confused with the question of whether you love them; they are not the same. If you are still struggling with whether to make the move, ask yourself these questions:

1. Do you see this relationship lasting in the long term?
2. In other circumstances, would you ever move to this city?
3. If this is a city where you would not otherwise go, will you take responsibility for the decision if things do not work out?
4. What conditions would have to be met before you would move there?

Every person will answer these questions differently. Here's how I answered them when I faced this decision:

1. Yes, I saw the relationship lasting in the long term (Spoiler alert: I was right. We're married.)
2. No, I would never move to Miami otherwise.
3. If the relationship doesn't work out or the city fails as a good fit, I will not resent Brian for it. I'm making an adult decision.
4. Before I move to Miami, I want to secure a job and apartment so that I can start to feel rooted and independent there.

The process of moving for a partner will undoubtedly be difficult — moving is awful even in the best circumstances. But by openly addressing the implications of the move up front, you can focus on the physical and not the emotional baggage.

Long-distance dating

During Brian's first year of medical school, I moved to Southeast Asia to teach and travel. That year, he lived in an anatomy lab and I gallivanted around Asia and taught small Thai children their ABCs. Not only were we both busy, but we were literally across the world from one another with a 12-hour time difference. We could not talk between the hours of 12:00 and 7:00 because one of us was always asleep.

Living in the same city (or on the same continent) is not an option for every couple. Some SOs choose not or cannot move for their med student partners, creating the unenviable long distance dating situation. Long-distance relationships are never easy, and adding medical school to the mix only magnifies the stress. Relationships grow when couples experience new things together and strengthen their emotional connection. Long-distance dating prevents the formation of new joint experiences as a couple, and often forces couples to focus on relationship maintenance rather than growth.

In these situations, new memories and emotional bonding are built during short visits. These visits are vital to the life of the relationship. In addition to spending time together and physically interacting, visits enable you to see where your partner lives, where they like to go, where they work, and who they spend time with. *Connect with the little details about their life.* There's immense power in being able to picture where your partner spends time and what your partner does each day. Before I moved to Asia, I visited Brian in Miami, where I met his friends and visited the medical school (a riveting experience, let me tell you). That visit created a vital link between me and Brian's day to day life. Unfortunately, Brian could not see what my life looked like in Bangkok. We initially struggled while I was away–Brian could not begin to fathom my day-to-day life and I struggled to paint that picture for him. That winter, Brian came to Thailand for one week. The visit saved our relationship. He saw where I slept, what I ate, and got a taste for Thai culture. We were back on even footing because we felt equally connected to one another's daily surroundings.

Infrequent visits come with added pressure to make each one feel extraordinary. The visits start to feel like a performance rather than time spent with a partner. My suggestion? Be ok with spending a weekend sitting on the couch, doing work, or going grocery shopping. Most of the experience of being in a relationship revolves around ordinary life. Certainly outings are important to your relationships, but so is seeing that you can cook dinner together.

Whether you decide to move for your partner or date long distance, establishing expectations and creating regular communication habits will be vital to the ongoing health of your relationship. Here are a few other suggestions for staying connected when you are apart:

Memorize each other's schedules: Do not just have each other's schedules, learn them. Memorize them. Be able to reference them. The more you know about one another's day-to-day life, the more connected you will feel.

Visit one another: Visit each other whenever possible (duh). This will help you stay connected to the people and intricacies in their life and help you feel less distant.

Do something "together": Create your own book club and read the same book at the same time. Watch the same TV series at the same pace (no Netflix cheating, people). Train for an athletic event that you will do together in person.

Learn the one-sentence method: Each of you write down one sentence about your day, each day. Email one another the statements at the end of the week. That way, even if you cannot talk every day, you will hear highlights and reference stories that you can ask about later.

Take up old-school letter writing: Mail each other handwritten letters. Like, with postage. Because so few people use letters to communicate, they can be meaningful way to connect.

CHAPTER 3
HOW IS DATING A MEDICAL STUDENT DIFFERENT?

"We come unbidden into this life, and if we are lucky we find a purpose beyond star-vation, misery, and early death which, lest we forget, is the common lot. I grew up and I found my purpose and it was to become a physician. My intent wasn't to save the world as much as to heal myself. Few doctors will admit this, certainly not young ones, but subconsciously, in entering the profession, we must believe that ministering to oth-ers will heal our woundedness. And it can. but it can also deepen the wound."
— *Abraham Verghese, Cutting for Stone*

While time commitment and financial trajectory questions apply to couples in a wide range of fields, the role of doctors in American culture, the length of training, the financial pressure, and the high stakes create a unique brand of stress. Understanding the combination of features in a medical career will inform the way you understand your partner's journey in med school.

Doctors hold an unusual place in American culture. They are skilled sci-entific clinicians who are well paid for their services and occupy a moral high ground for their work helping sick and injured people. This rare combina-tion makes others look up to and respect doctors for their knowledge and expertise. Even their attire is special. A physician's white coat signals compe-tence. Doctors adopted the white coat in the mid-19th century to lend them the credibility of laboratory workers who sported them. The color white was chosen to associate physicians with purity and cleanliness. With a few excep-tions, patients want their doctors to wear white coats, reporting that it con-fers confidence in the doctor's abilities, improves communication, and fosters the doctor-patient relationship.[2]

---

2   Miles Landry, et al., "Patient Preferences for Doctor Attire: The White Coat's Place in the

Dating a medical student means dating somebody soon to be at the top of the prestige hierarchy. Doctors rank highly on the official Jewish Bubbes' List of Acceptable Jobs for My Grandchild. (The list is released annually, but Doctor has been in the top slot for 347 years in a row.) You are likely to encounter comments that focus on the prestige of becoming a doctor. In reaction to mentioning your partner's status as a medical student, you may encounter raised eyebrows, impressed nods, and compliments about your partner's ambition, drive, intelligence, and altruism. One SO described the phenomenon this way: "Everybody is impressed. 'OMG a [doctor] at an impressive school.' People are preposterously impressed." Dating somebody in this prestigious field means receiving judgements and comments about their choices.

Many hold doctors to a higher moral standard, expecting them to treat their profession as a calling — an altruistic undertaking for the good of mankind, divorced from ambition and financial, professional, and cultural expectations. While some doctors view medicine as a calling, many do not. Law students and PhD candidates less commonly bear the same expectations to view their career track in such a selfless way. This pedestal phenomenon creates additional stress.

Because of the way society views doctors, others will make assumptions about how you will live your life. People in your life may assume that your collective life trajectory revolves around medicine. In lieu of what people see as imminent financial stability and prestige, those around you may fail to ask you about your career choice or assume that you will work only if it is financially necessary. Many SOs encounter an engrained assumption that the medical career is more important than yours, or that your career trajectory should take a back seat to your med student's. This can be a stressful corollary to the pride you feel about your partner's career.

I have experienced this attitude many times. During our honeymoon, Brian and I were walking with an older couple with whom we had become friendly. The man asked Brian where we were from and what he did. Brian explained that we were moving to Philadelphia after the honeymoon and that he was starting residency. Without missing a beat, the man looks at me and

Medical Profession," *The Ochsner Journal* 13, no. 3 (2013).

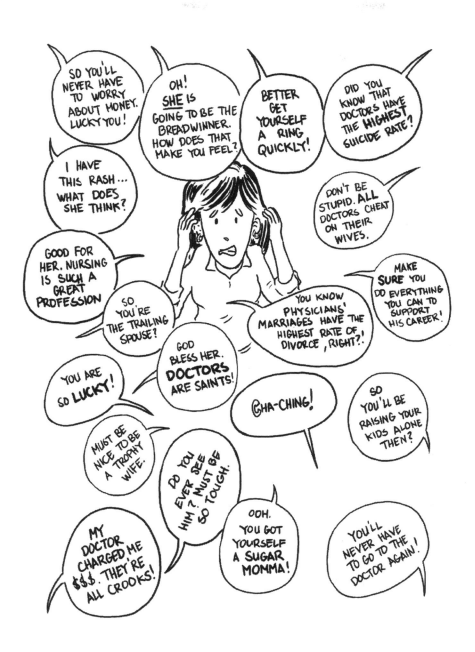

says, "Ah, so you are the trailing spouse?" He didn't ask about my career or choices. Instead, he voiced the common assumption that our lives revolved around Brian's medical career.

It takes almost forever to become a doctor. OK, not actually forever, but it certainly feels like it. Medical school lasts four years, followed by a three- to seven-year residency, and possible fellowships after that. Law school and business school take three years each. PhDs may take as long as medical school, but they often come with a stipend (though often paltry) that can help keep students from accruing extensive student loan debt. The number of years it takes a person to become a doctor presents individual and relationship challenges related to financial planning, location, identity, and work life that can wear on a relationship. A couple must stay in a particular city for four years, which limits your options. Many SOs are in their twenties, exploring their careers, planning their futures, and looking at graduate school. In serious relationships, the financial cost also impacts both parties in the relationship. The four years spent not earning an income, the delayed nest-egg building, and the daunting task of paying off debt all must be accepted as the realities of dating a medical student, most of the time.

These distinct features present both advantages and challenges. On the bright side, doctors enjoy respect, status, and clinical prowess. Once practicing as physicians, they can expect a relatively high standard of living. It feels good to provide tangible evidence of helping other human beings. On the other hand, training for a job with such high stakes creates immense stress on medical students and their relationships.

So, fine: Doctors are different. But you are not dating a doctor; you are dating a medical student. And that is a vital distinction, because the stressors for doctors and medical students are not always the same. Yes, loans bring stress, but not as the primary stressor during school. Yes, doctors end up on a pedestal, and you should remain aware of that. But within the profession, medical students huddle at the bottom of the totem pole. While these are the big picture realities, the educational barriers account for the majority of a student's stress.

Institutional pressures

When discussing medical students, some write off the stress as being the result of what happens to an inherently high-strung bunch, predisposed to struggle with mental health. That is a myth. When they enter medical school, med students have a similar or better level of mental health than their fellow college graduates. Well-equipped and experienced in managing difficult workloads, medical students' mental health nevertheless drops below that of their non-medical classmates when they enter school.[3] It can be hard to understand the exact source of the pressure. Are medical students putting all the pressure on themselves? Are the classes really that competitive? A combination of institutional and personal factors forms the stress that medical students face.

The grading system

For example, how your partner's medical school grades students influences how stressed your partner gets, particularly during their first year of school. Medical schools with a steep grading structure — meaning letter grades rather than a pass/fail system — exacerbate the stress, recording a 1.97 times higher rate of student burnout, which makes the transition into medical school more difficult.[4] Schools using a pass/fail grading system, in contrast, help students ease into their new environment and develop support systems that increase resilience.

On top of normal stressors, female medical students encounter several additional stressors during their training. In terms of gender makeup of medical school classes, schools worldwide reached gender parity in 2003,[4] and by 2005 medical school classes were 60 percent women and 40 percent men.[5] Unfortunately, women face difficulties breaking into this historically male

3   Liselotte Dyrbye and Tait Shanafelt, "A narrative review on burnout experienced by medical students and residents," *Medical Education* 50, no. 1 (2015): , doi:10.1111/medu.12927.
4   Barbara Buddeberg-Fischer et al., "The impact of gender and parenthood on physicians' careers - professional and personal situation seven years after graduation," *BMC Health Services Research* 10, no. 1 (2010): , doi:10.1186/1472-6963-10-40.
5   Alan Bleakley, "Gender matters in medical education," *Medical Education* 47, no. 1 (2012): , doi:10.1111/j.1365-2923.2012.04351.x.

profession. Women will struggle to find mentorship in medicine because most medical faculty members are men. Women are under-represented in leadership positions, and at the current rate of growth, it will take 25 years for women to attain even half the proportion of full professorship positions that men currently hold in medical schools. Leaders model career trajectory and show us that we belong. If a department has only tall white men on faculty, it makes others feel like they do not belong.

Women in medical school and medicine more commonly face sexism and comments that undermine their authority in clinical spaces. Many scrub companies do not make scrubs and white coats for petite women, sending the message that petite women do not belong. Women encounter criticism for their appearance or can be penalized for showing empathy and caring because this implies less efficiency or competence. Every one of my female medical student friends regularly gets called "Nurse." Older male patients may treat female medical students paternalistically, and some have been told that they are "too pretty" or "too young" to be a doctor.[6] A hospital maintenance worker told one of my female physician friends to "smile," and another petite female physician friend was told by an old male patient that she must be "this tall" (indicating taller than her 5 feet) to be a doctor. For partners of female medical students, these very real systemic issues create stress and frustration. As their partner, your job includes knowing that they are not making it up, they are not exaggerating, and that this is deeply entrenched in medical culture. Female partners of female medical students may find it easier to relate, but male partners also must be fully supportive when these instances arise.

The competition for residency

Still, it can also feel like their stress is overblown. Of course the material is hard! But they'll be fine — they already got into medical school. They just need to get through, right? Well, maybe. To practice medicine, students must first get into medical residencies (paid training positions for new doctors)

---

6   Gail Erlick Robinson, "Stresses on women physicians: Consequences and coping techniques," *Depression and Anxiety* 17, no. 3 (2003): , doi:10.1002/da.10069.

after med school ends. Students apply during their fourth year of medical school and residency programs take a limited number of residents in each medical specialty. That number is determined by the hospital's capacity and federal funding to pay the physician residents. In 1997, Congress passed the Balanced Budget Act, which enabled Medicare to providing funding to offset the costs of educating residents. That is a good thing. Unfortunately, Congress set a fixed number of funded spots in 1997 and never increased it. Meanwhile, the population grew, patient care got more complicated, and the government encouraged medical schools to take on more medical students to address a growing doctor shortage.[7] So, they did! In fact, medical schools are on target to increase classes by 30 percent by 2019,[8] to say nothing of new medical schools that are opening. *But wait,* you might be thinking, *adding more students to medical schools without increasing the number of residency spots does not solve the doctor shortage problem.* You are correct! As of early 2017, congress is creating more residency spots, but the numbers are still tight. Lobby your congressperson through the American Medical Association (AMA)'s advocacy branch, located at ama-assn.org. Then bang your head against a wall in frustration.

Further complicating the issue, prestigious programs and attractive cities and specialties receive disproportionate applications, making the process that much more competitive. Many residencies are located in cities, towns, and rural areas where most people do not want to live. So, many students with competitive school grades and scores find the increased competition forces them to apply to residency programs in places that house more cows than students. The fear of not matching combined with the fear of matching in an undesirable location sits in the back of medical student's mind. It is the fearful mantra undergirding every late-night study session and missed date.

---

7   Rich Daly, "AAMC Issues Alert About Looming Physician Shortage," *Psychiatric News* 44, no. 2 (2009): , doi:10.1176/pn.44.2.0004a.
8   "Medical School Enrollment to Approach 30 Percent Increase by 2019," Association of American Medical Colleges, accessed May 09, 2017, https://www.aamc.org/newsroom/news-releases/431036/20150430.html.

The financial stress

While we're talking about institutionalized stressors, let's briefly look at medical students' financial trajectory. Here is a snapshot: According to the Association of American Medical Colleges' 2016 "Debt, Costs, and Loan Repayment Fact Card" 76% of medical students graduate an average of $189,165 and go on to make $53,580 as a first year resident. Throughout residency, the interest on the debt accrues at roughly 6.8 percent for the average student loan. In addition to those growing burdens, med students give up the earnings that they would have earned if they started working right out of undergrad. While often viewed as the path to wealth, that path gets ever harder to navigate.

For couples, the financial stress can manifest in both the long and short term. In the short term, students are often strapped for cash. In the long term, couples must find different ways to plan to buy a home, have children, and travel. For relationships with long-term ambitions, the question lingers of how to accommodate medical training and other expensive investments made during a person's twenties and thirties. Medical couples must adopt an alternative financial plan that considers the priorities of loan repayment and stalled next steps, with the knowledge that eventually, physicians generally make a comfortable living. We will talk in Chapter 6 about how to address finances and I will give you resources to help you get started.

The impact of institutional stress

So, given the career and institutional stress, students manage a great deal of emotional strain. The trope is familiar — overachievers are shocked when they find themselves surrounded by all the other smartest kids in the class. The extreme competition in medical school classes filled with overachievers can quickly start to impact the students' self-esteem. For many, achievement is a central tenet of identity. One SO talked about starting medical school this way: "He had emotional changes that I didn't necessarily understand. ... All the sudden, he had to let go of that idea in his mind of being the top of his class." Another talked about watching the "emotional drain it can have on a person psychologically for students who do not necessarily have an easy time in school," citing her partner's past struggles in school and new levels of competition. Students whose self-worth relies on achievement can struggle to acclimate to new barometers of success. Your partner may start to think and say things like:

- I am not studying enough; everybody else studies more than I do.
- I am not as smart as my classmates.
- I must be the only one who doesn't understand this lecture.
- How am I going to keep up?

Understanding depression and treatment for medical students

Given the institutional stressors, it should come as no surprise to hear that medical students experience higher rates of depression than the general population, with progressively worse mental health over the course of medical training. Unfortunately, medical students are far less likely than the general public to seek and receive treatment because they face the infuriating, *no-seriously-this-is-still-a-thing?* irony that medical students and medical schools view mental illness as a weakness. Students worry that seeking treatment will go into their record and residencies will be less likely to hire them. These fears, unfortunately, may not be unfounded. In one study, residency directors said they were less likely to ask a hypothetical applicant to interview if they had any history of receiving psychological counseling. Some state medical boards may require students to disclose a history of depression, meet with a psychiatrist, or get a report from the applicant's physician. Thirty-seven percent of students cited the lack of confidentiality and 24 percent cited fear of documentation as the reason they would not seek treatment. [9]

Very quickly, depression can lead to burnout, and indeed, medical students experience high levels of burnout, meaning emotional exhaustion, cynicism, and a low sense of personal accomplishment. After adjusting for age, sex, relationship status, and hours worked per week, medical students

9 Rosenthal, Julie M., and Susan Okie, "White Coat, Mood Indigo — Depression in Medical School," *New England Journal of Medicine 353, no. 11* (2005): , doi:10.1056/nejmp058183.

suffer a higher risk for burnout than those with a bachelor's degree, master's degree, or other doctoral level degrees such as a JD or PhD! Worse, by the time medical students graduate, the typical burnout rate is 49 percent. What causes these high rates of burnout? For first- and second-years, it is correlated to having less supportive faculty and staff and a dissatisfying learning environment. Third year and fourth year students attribute their burnout to "the overall learning environment, poor clerkship organization, and working with cynical residents."[10]

In response to ever-increasing levels of stress, medical students adapt, often by adopting unhealthy coping mechanisms. In his book, *Doctors' Marriages*, Michael Myers includes an apt description of medical students' burnout response. He writes,

> They acclimate to toxic environments and ways of managing stresses rather than changing things so that life is lived in a more self-nurturing manner. In short, they confuse the concepts of noble and normal. Wealth of coping strength actually pre-disposes you to making a fundamental stress-management mistake: because of your exceptional coping abilities, you are at risk of normalizing what is essentially an abnormal way of living; no matter how stressed you get, you are capable of going numb and pressing on.[11]

While some stress is inevitable, burnout is not. Because many medical schools do not provide tools to prevent or help with burnout, medical students and their partners often manage these psychological realities on their own. There are proven ways to reduce burnout and maintain mental health while in medical school, and, as it turns out, they are the same things that can help create a healthy relationship (go figure). The topic of increasing med student access to mental healthcare and creating institutional changes that pro-

---

10   Dyrbye, Lisolette, and Tait Shanafelt, T. (2015). A narrative review on burnout experienced by medical students and residents. *Medical Education,* 50, no. 1 (2015): 132-149. doi:10.1111/medu.12927.
11   Michael F. Myers, *Doctors' Marriages: A look at the problems and their solutions* (New York, NY: Plenum Medical Books, 1988).

mote medical student wellbeing, abound. While I will not go into in-depth descriptions of these topics, I included a burnout section in the resource list at the end of the book.

CHAPTER 4
UNIQUE STRESSORS YOU MAY FACE

"And when the event, the big change in your life, is simply an insight — isn't that a strange thing? That absolutely nothing changes except that you see things differently and you are less fearful and less anxious and generally stronger as a result: isn't it amazing that a completely invisible thing in your head can feel realer than anything you've experienced before?"
— Jonathan Franzen, *The Corrections*

The important (and obvious) next question is, what about you? What are the unique stressors you should expect as the partner of a medical student?

Lopsided emotional support

Every relationship has three entities that want attention, love, and support: you, your partner, and the relationship itself. Every couple's task is to balance the needs of all three entities. When that support falls to one member of the couple, they may start to feel taken advantage of, lonely, hurt, or resentful. Medical couples risk falling into a pattern that asks you, the non-medical student, to ensure the ongoing health of the relationship while also emotionally supporting both yourself and your partner. Your partner may ask you to listen to them vent about their stressors, seek your help studying, or ask you to give them space to work. If you live with your partner, they may ask you to take on more domestic responsibilities to accommodate their academic needs. You may have to answer to mutual friends who ask why your partner cannot (or can never!) hang out. While you take on the additional responsibilities of helping your partner manage growing stress, they may feel unable to emulate that level of support for you. If you're aware of these dynamics, you can manage them, find ways to mitigate them, and restore the balance of responsibility at different points throughout school.

You may have to carry your stress, as well as theirs and the relationship's, for long periods of time. Social worker and medical spouse Jordyn Hagar, in her book *At Least You will be Married to a Doctor,* calls this concept "one-sided emotion work." She defines one-sided emotion work as occurring when

> One member of the relationship is primarily the giver and the other is primarily the receiver. ... It means that more frequently you will find yourself actively supporting your partner and his emotional experience than [they] will be actively supporting you and your emotional experience.[12]

To address and minimize the imbalance you will want to do three things. First, notice it. Become a researcher in your life and relationship. Notice the balance of emotional support, when it gets lopsided, and what contributes to the imbalance. Are they asking for too much? Are you offering more than you can give when you are already busy? Both may be factors. Watch for patterns that emerge. Do you pick up the slack when your partner studies but struggle to regain balance when an exam ends and they have more time to commit to the relationship? Do you and your partner find ways to nurture the relationship during stressful periods? Do you find yourself failing to address issues because medical school always feels more urgent and important? These kinds of dynamics commonly emerge and continue until somebody notices them. Try to approach the practice of noticing without judgment of yourself or your partner. Watching the dynamics unfurl with curiosity rather than judgment can make addressing and shifting them a collaborative rather than adversarial activity. Here are a few phrases that can help guide your self-research:
- I notice that when my partner does _____, I do _____.
- When I ask for _____, I receive _____.
- I am grateful when my partner does _____ for me.

---

12 Jordyn Paradis Hagar, *At least you'll be married to a doctor: Managing your intimate relationship through medical school* (Denver, CO: Outskirts Press, 2012).

- I most need emotional support during _____ times.
- Before an exam, I notice that we fall into the pattern of _____.

Once you notice the dynamics, you can start to address them as a team. Once again, try to focus on non-judgment and curiosity and discuss things that feel unfair as a joint task for the two of you to address together. If you feel like you aren't receiving enough acknowledgement — ask for it. If they mention that they need more moral support when they are studying, hear them. Once you've talked about what you noticed and perhaps what they noticed, set a time to check in, in a month to see how things are going. Give yourselves time to learn new habits and patterns.

Finally, develop your own emotional support system because realistically, you will encounter times when you need support and your partner cannot provide it.

Medicine: the third member of your relationship

Remember how I said that a med school partner can start to feel like a third wheel in a two-person relationship? Well, let's take that idea a step further. Think of medical school as a member of your relationship. When you and your partner sit in a room together to discuss your priorities, it sits in the room too, putting in its two cents and demanding you both adhere to its power over everybody else. Thinking of medical school as a distinct entity that throws its weight around will you see the demands coming from the school, not the student. As an external party, the two of you can address its needs while still holding the student responsible for their role in the relationship. Your partner has committed to a relationship with medical school, and in choosing to date them, you agree to medical school having a say in the room.

Envy and comparing life tracks

Despite the arduous journey, medical school provides its trainees with a clear path toward a lucrative, well-respected, mapped-out career. While these features may foster a sense of safety and pride, if you are working a first job that you do not love, applying to school, or still figuring things out, your partner's stability and certainty may lead you to feel insecure, envious, or stressed out. Few career paths are as mapped out as a medical career; medicine tells students where to go, what to study, and how to reach the next step on the career ladder. Most of us follow career trajectories that zigzag and veer based on our credentials, connections, the economy, and luck.

Watch out for envy that may emerge from watching your partner progress through medical school. Envy may be masking your own fear — you may be scared about where your own career is going or comparing dissimilar career paths. That fear makes sense. Try focusing on you and what you want from your life as one way to ease the pressures of your med student's path. Separate yourself in your mind. You are not in competition and your paths will not look the same, even if you are both medical students!

HOW IT CAN FEEL COMPARING YOUR LIFE TRAJECTORY TO A MED LIFE TRAJECTORY

If you want to share that fear with your partner, focus the observation on your vulnerability rather than how stable their career path feels to you. If you approach your partner and say, "It is so unfair that you do not have to worry about what you will do next. You just apply to residency and you are set," they may feel defensive when you're seeking support and feel less able to address the way you feel. They may start listing all the reasons their path is stressful, turning the conversation into a stress competition. Instead, try saying something like, "I'm feeling really scared about the next step in my career. It scares me that I cannot see what I want in long term."

Some may find that their partner does not understand the struggles related to finding one's career or life path. Many med students chose this path as children and never strayed. If this description sounds familiar to you, be aware that they may not understand the notion that not everybody figures out what they want at a young age. Those partners who feel confident in their own long-term goals, either in school, working a job they loved, or raising children, better manage the med school have more emotional energy to bear its demands.

Competitive stress

You and your partner each walk through the door after a long day. Feeling overwhelmed by a long day at the office, at school, or running errands, you start telling your partner about your day. Your partner, home from an exam, a full day of class, a long rotation, or a yucky day dissecting a cadaver, feels stressed and overwhelmed and wants to tell you about it. In fact, after you lay out why you are stressed, they counter with their own frustrations. Thinking they do not understand just how bad your day was, you emphasize some of the more salient points of your day. They counter with how many hours they still have to study tonight. The process continues and you both grow frustrated. An opportunity to connect just morphed into a spitting contest over whose day was worse.

Many couples stumble into stress competitions when both people's lives are hectic. Each person wants empathy and support, but neither provides it. Instead of seeing two distinct stories that each deserve empathy, you begin comparing them as if only one of you deserves the empathy that comes from enduring a difficult day. Competitive stress needlessly turns validation into a zero-sum game.

The good news? You and your partner can catch this dynamic as it unfurls and nip it in the bud. The moment you each start talking about your own stressors without responding to your partner's, pause. Notice that you each feel unfulfilled. Then, break your interaction into two separate conversations. You might say, "I do want to hear about your day and your studying. Before we do that, could I tell you about my rough day? I need to vent and I do not want us to compete over whose day was worse." You might even point out what's happening as it happens: "I think we're doing that thing again where we are both eager to vent but we're basically trying to one-up each other. Why don't you tell me what happened in class and then can I tell you what happened at work?" This way, each person gets the chance to talk about their day, and neither person's stress receives a more coveted slot.

Sometimes, competitive stress emerges when two people feel stressed out about the same event or stressor. Medical school can easily become a topic that creates mutual stress and leads a couple to fight over who maintains a right to that stress. As we've discussed, medical school can feel rightfully stressful for both you and your partner. While their stress may tie to their immediate responsibilities, yours might tie to the health of the relationship or the long-term implications of their performance in school. On some days, Brian stressed about the outcomes of his exams and rotations. On other days, the impact that medical school would have on our future felt truly overwhelming to me. Sometimes, we felt stressed about medical school at the same time. When that happened, it was hard to step back and validate one another's concerns without trying to elevate our own. It took a conscious effort to create two separate conversations. But learning to separate our conversations ultimately helped each of us feel supported and heard.

The reality: dealing with absence

An SO I spoke to described dating a medical student with a single word: "absence." Another talked about an exponential decrease in the number of conversations, stories, and experiences that they and their partner shared. Still another SO described their marriage to a med student this way: "It is like being married to the shadow of a person. You are married to the idea of a person." In fact, almost every SO I spoke to mentioned the lack of time together as a major obstacle to maintaining a healthy relationship. Over long periods of time, hours of absence can wreak havoc on a relationship, growing the risk of living parallel lives. The Sotile Center for Physician Resilience echoes this sentiment, consistently showing in its research that the biggest source of conflict in medical marriages is a lack of time for fun, the family, and the self.[13] Further, planning becomes nearly impossible because the student often cannot predict exactly how much study time they will need and they do not set their own clinical hours.

Spending time alone and loneliness

As a result of their absence, partners of medical students spend lots of time alone. You will attend social events, weddings, and dinners alone. You are likely to do weekend travel alone. Sometimes your partner may be home but unavailable to spend time together, physically there but mentally absent. Your partner may want to spend some precious free time with friends, catching up on hobbies, and calling family members. You will feel like you want to hog them, but sometimes you cannot. You may feel like you need them while they feel pulled in multiple directions by others who also want their attention. For this reason, SOs who depend solely on their partner for social and emotional fulfillment will struggle, because med students cannot do that for them.

The dread of waiting

If you do not plan for time alone, you may inadvertently find yourself becoming resentful while waiting for your partner to stop studying and pay attention to you. When I asked SOs what advice they would give others dating

---

13   Sotile, Wayne M., and Mary O. Sotile. "Physicians' wives evaluate their marriages, their husbands, and life in medicine: Results of the AMA-Alliance Medical Marriage Survey.", *Bulletin of the Menninger Clinic*, vol. 68, no. 1 (2004) 39–59. doi:10.1521/bumc.68.1.39.27730.

medical students, *every single person* told me a variation of "do not sit at home and wait for them." Many told me that the most difficult times during medical school occurred when their medical student partner was swamped and they had a lot of free time.

Grief for the loss of a "normal" life

When I started dating Brian, I had no inkling that by dedicating myself to a medical student, I was forfeiting some of the expectations I held for my life. We would never live a "normal" life because his working hours would never be 9 to 5, and days off would not necessarily align with weekends. I felt disoriented by the sense that I wrote my life's story and looked up to discover another reality entirely. I did not realize that until he finished residency, almost every month would mean a new rotation with a different schedule, different colleagues, and different expectations. As our lives melded into one shared life, I began to grieve the loss of that "normal" life, the life I originally foresaw for myself. As Hagar points out in her book *At Least You will be Married to a Doctor*,

"Universally, significant others of med students tend to grieve, to some extent or another, for the life that we had thought we would have before med school entered our lives. … We just all lost the vision of a life without medicine."

For many, this grief also gives rise to loneliness or self-judgement about feeling bad. Friends and family may struggle to empathize because your struggle is tied to something others envy or see as an objectively good outcome (being with a future doctor). You may feel angry at yourself for struggling with the burden of this new path. I am here to tell you that it is OK to grieve. It is OK to feel sad that your life may not look the way you thought it would. You can even grieve if you feel grateful and happy with your current life.

Grief unexamined and left unaddressed can morph into its ugly step-cousin, resentment. Resentment is tricky because it seems to burrow itself into your brain. While grief can feel like a sharp penetrating pain, resentment seethes and may only emerge when a sore point gets (metaphorically) poked with a stick. Even worse, resenting medicine means resenting a nontangible entity. You cannot yell at medical school, curse at medical school, and angrily step on medical school's big toe. You cannot tell medical school to stop asking for so much money, time, and emotional energy. You cannot tell medical school that you need your partner's attention and affection because you had a bad day or your grandmother just died. Medical school is omnipresent but silent, remember? It sits in your room and wordlessly makes its demands known. The only person who can respond to your resentment about medical school is your partner.

Coming out of grief by writing a new story

How do we examine and overcome the grief we feel about this unexpected life turn? When you are ready, you will write yourself a new narrative. We all tell stories about the trajectory of our lives. When something unexpected happens, part of the healing process involves weaving that episode into your story. In our life's narrative, we may describe a lost opportunity as a turning point that led to other opportunities. Random encounters may be told as a destined meeting. Getting fired becomes the best thing that ever happened to us, because it made us realize what we really wanted. We come to terms with death by describing it as the peaceful ending to a well-lived life. Our lives are Play-Doh — ours to shape and harden however we see fit. We have all met people who choose to interpret every event in a negative light. We have also all met that person who seems to seamlessly integrate adversity and life's curve balls into their personal narrative. How we tell our story can determine whether we proceed feeling resentment, pride, happiness, or resignation. Your life took a different, unexpected turn when you became committed to a medical student? OK. Now how are you going to tell the story about your life?

I spent three years living in Miami so that I could be near Brian while he finished med school. During that time, I worked in for-profit marketing and then nonprofit project management. I struggled, I was frequently unhappy, and I lost a few jobs along the way. When we left Miami, I wondered how I should think about those years. They did not contribute to my current career path (unless you count this book). For a long time, I wondered if I would have to live with the burden of feeling like those were wasted years. I spent months processing that period, which felt so out of place in my otherwise tidy, successful life. People tried to help. They told me that it was all worth it because in the end, I had Brian. But that narrative did not resonate. That way of interpreting my time in Miami did not jive with how I saw myself.

I now believe that I would have struggled in some form or another in my early twenties. That narrative makes me feel OK about the struggles I underwent during those years. If I'd been even moderately happy doing marketing work, I never would have had the courage to apply to graduate school in couple and family therapy, a decision that has made me exceptionally happy. I never would have started writing this book. There are lots of ways to interpret an experience and this interpretation gave me control over my story. Could I choose to view it as wasted time? Sure. But I am much happier thinking about my life in this way. The important thing is to examine your grief and fit it into your story. Every story is different. What's yours?

CHAPTER 5
UNDERSTANDING MED SCHOOL'S
TIME STRUCTURE

"Many people think that the secret to reconnecting with their partner is a candlelit dinner or a by-the-sea vacation. The real secret is to turn toward each other in the little ways every day."
— John Gottman, *The Seven Principles for Making Marriage Work*

No one solution can solve the lack of time you get to spend with your partner. But understanding medical school's trajectory, avoiding some common pitfalls, embracing flexibility, and building other supports will make your life easier. To get started, let's talk about how medical school plays out and how it will impact the way you structure your life and your relationship. Each school's timing differs a little, so try to learn that information far in advance so you can plan. But this outline will be mostly accurate for most students.

Structural overview of medical school

Medical school requires four years of study. Not unlike the first two years of any graduate school program, first and second year medical students attend lectures, labs, and discussion groups on topics such as anatomy, microbiology, and physiology, taking periodic exams. As one SO put it, "First and second year are awful but predictable." At the end of second year, medical students take Step 1, the first part of a three-part medical licensing examination series (more in Chapter 7). During third and fourth year, medical students do clinical rotations full-time in clinics and hospitals. Many rotations (generally between 2 and 12 weeks long) include an exam at the end. At the end of third year or in the middle of fourth year, students take Step 2 of the medical boards. During fourth year, medical students apply to medical residencies in their chosen specialty. The interview process takes place throughout the fall and part of the spring, and students find out their residency assignments in mid-March. Students graduate in May of their fourth year.

Big picture

By the time your partner is an attending physician (meaning they have completed all their training), medical training can dictate a decade or more of a person's decisions and movements. A student spends four years accruing pre-med credits during their undergraduate career, followed by four years of medical school, three-seven years in residency, and an option one-three years of fellowship for those becoming specialists. This timeline only accounts for the most direct path to a medical degree. Many students take training detours, such as:

Post baccalaureate training:

If a student completes college without taking required pre-med courses and waits to go to med school, they will need one or two years to complete those prerequisites.

Before and during medical school:

Many students take a year (or more) off between undergraduate and medical school to conduct research, complete their applications, earn another degree, or even (gasp!) work in the real world. Some students take a year off during med school to conduct research to bolster their residency application, particularly if they plan to apply to a competitive specialty.

Additional degrees:

Still other students enter MD/PhD programs, which are structured with the four-five year PhD program sandwiched between the second and third year of medical school. Others work toward an MD/MPH (Master of Publish Health), MD/MBA (Master of Business Administration), or another dual de-

CHALLENGE: NOT MAKING MEDICINE
THE SCAPEGOAT FOR EVERY
RELATIONSHIP ISSUE

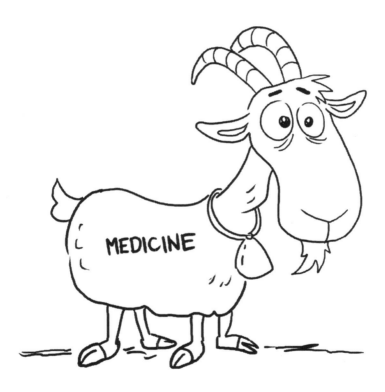

gree. These generally add one or two years. (Osteopathic students can substitute DO for the MD here — it works the same.)

There are dozens of potential reasons to take time off before, during, and after medical school. Brian had a classmate who took a year off in the middle of medical school to pursue his professional racecar-driving career (medicine was his backup plan).

A person pursuing a career in medicine has likely internalized the length and implications of this timeline. It is time for you to start thinking about it because committing to a med student means committing to their timeline. This timeline controls a med student's location and choices for many years, and you will not be immune from its effects. *Your* career, movement, and decisions will be impacted. Medical school often coincides with a valuable chunk of career development years. If your partner starts medical school at 23, for example, and you choose to live near them, you commit to turning down opportunities in other locations. You commit to potentially living in a place that lacks the resources and infrastructure needed to reach your goals. You may need to get creative about your planning. On the other side, you may get settled during medical school and then have to uproot for residency.

The postponement trap

Sometimes medical school gets prioritized over your relationship's immediate needs, making it difficult to figure out when you should advocate for time together, or time for yourself and the relationship. Medical school always feels more urgent than your relationship, but allowing the relationship to take a back seat completely will not solve the problem.

If you constantly put off your and your relationship's problems in deference to medical school's urgency, you may join the ranks of medical couples that allow medical school to become the scapegoat. Both partners, and particularly the student's significant other, embrace the psychology of postponement, becoming experts at delayed gratification.[14] The philosophy of work

---

14   Glen O. Gabbard and Roy W. Menninger, *Medical Marriages* (Washington, DC: American Psychiatric Press, 1988).

now, play later becomes a mantra that comes back to bite the couple later on. Medical couples grow used to "a life of waiting," hoping they get around to enjoying life and the relationship after finishing medical school.[15] This may manifest in thoughts such as: "When medical school is over, we'll go on that vacation we keep putting off," or, "When medical school is over, we'll get into a better place in our relationship where it feels more equal and satisfying."

On the one hand, relying on postponement makes sense and provides a natural response to having very little time with a partner. It helps stave off disappointment and resentment. You will have to postpone certain things to accommodate medical school, and coping with that reality can be eased when you remind yourself that medical school is temporary and that you will be able to do "it" later. We're even taught as children that delaying gratification signals maturity; kids want the cookie and they want it now; adults can say no to the cookie for the sake of the health benefits later. (I'm more of a cookie girl, myself, but perhaps that is part of the problem…) On the other hand, with medical school as a worthy scapegoat, you do not want to wake up in 10 years and find that you've lost the chance to do things you wanted to do.

The concept of postponement is complex; sometimes conversations do need to be put off while your partner studies for an exam or finishes a particularly exhausting rotation. That said, the dirty underside of postponement is that medical couples use it to avoid important conversations and fights. The mindset of postponement enables unhappy partners to avoid their relationship anxiety and put off dealing with problems. A reason to postpone a tough conversation always exists. But it is important to approach every situation individually rather than use medical school as a blanket excuse not to address issues. Do not let "we'll deal with it later" become a crutch or a mantra.

Pros and cons aside, postponement as a plan will not work. When they finish medical school, medical students become busier. They take on additional responsibilities, not fewer. Even after their training ends and they are making a decent salary, many doctors work many hours. Instead of viewing the medical lifestyle as a temporary hindrance, think about it as a lifestyle you

15   Wayne M. Sotile and Mary O. Sotile, *Medical Marriage: A couple's survival guide* (Scaucus, NJ: Carol Publishing Group, 1996).

are accepting and work around it and with it.

Postponement essentially invites death by 1,000 paper cuts. Relationships end up with tiny, unresolved issues. Dinner plans get canceled, partners do not find ways to spend time together, they miss opportunities to exchange affection. Each instance feels too insignificant to mention. But in aggregate, they add up and cannot be ignored. A medical student's partner often feels guilty complaining, or feels inadequate for not being self-sufficient. But ultimately, relationships evolve from tiny moments and finding ways to meet each other's needs.

Three steps to overcoming the time issue

But the problem persists: What do we do? It might be that you cannot have your or the relationship's needs fulfilled exactly when or how you'd like them addressed. You will both need to be flexible and amenable to creative solutions that require extra effort. Still, you can make it work, and successful medical couples share three basic habits that enable them to make the most of their limited schedules. They consistently:

1. Decide to prioritize one another
2. Make time during hectic lives
3. Negotiate on an ongoing basis

These three principles, straightforward as they sound, have been shown to insulate the couple during demanding stretches of time. Couples who do those three things have built themselves a foundation of regular communication and affection that enables them to feel safe and secure even when they cannot spend much time together.[16]

1. Decide

The first principle, deciding to prioritize one another, is both the easiest and the hardest. This one simply requires ongoing mental effort and an ongoing decision to commit yourself to the task of making time for your relation-

---

16 C. O. Fider, C. A. Fox, and C. M. Wilson, "Physicians in Dual-Career Marriages: Nurturing Their Relationships," *The Family Journal* 22, no. 4 (2014): , doi:10.1177/1066480714547699.

ship. Sometimes, that will feel easy. At other times, this will require immense mental and emotional energy. Over time, this can become a positive habit that you seamlessly integrate into your routine.

2. Make time

Making time during your hectic life together will always be complicated, but it can be made easier by employing some helpful strategies.

Swap schedules: Share your daily schedules with each other. Google Calendar has been a savior for many medical couples looking to coordinate. Put your schedules on the fridge and cross-reference them to find magical moments of free time. Having each other's schedule also helps you stay connected to one another's separate lives, a key to feeling connected when you are physically apart.

Think small and take study breaks: One SO put it this way. "Be OK with going out for coffee. That is something that [my partner] and I have done for the last 5 years, and that has been extremely helpful. You may not have a 5-hour break, but anybody can take a 25-minute coffee break." During study weeks leading up to exams, make it a point to eat dinner together. Everybody eats, and even if your partner only has 10 or 20 minutes, the break will give you both the chance to talk and unwind a little.

Enjoy the ebb: While medical school is always busy, *it does ebb and flow.* During first and second year, the ebb often comes at the beginning of units, before a student must study in earnest for an upcoming exam. Take advantage and go on a date! During third and fourth year, ebbs take place during lighter rotations. Plan to spend more time together during those lighter times.

Take advantage of technology: Take the time to send a cute or sexy message to your partner. Those messages show that you are making time for them even when you are not together.

Master the one-sentence method: Remember this trick from the long-distance section? Each write down one sentence about your day, each day. Email one another the statements at the end of the week. That way, even if you cannot talk every day, you will hear highlights and reference stories that you can ask about later.

Send snail mail: This tip, too. Even if you live together, buy cards for one another and leave each other handwritten notes.

More small gestures

Are you noticing a pattern? These strategies do not focus on big gestures. The strategies we listed reference simple tactics and mindsets to help you maximize your time together. Infusing your relationship with micro-doses of affection can help your relationship regardless of how much time you have to spend together. Small gestures of affection also stave off resentment and frustration and keep the relationship afloat during difficult stretches. They remind you and your partner that you matter to one another and that your relationship matters. When talking to SOs about what helped them get through medical school, many mentioned "think small" moments that they employed Here are some of their examples:

- A med student cooks dinner once a month and says they wish they could cook more often
- A med student takes on more household chores when faced with lighter studying
- A med student involves partner in studying
- A couple forms a communication agreements for when one partner has a long shift at the hospital. The med student sends a text once a day checking in, asking after their partner, or just saying that they are thinking about them
- Couple leaves one another notes on a mirror or cards on each other's pillows

How can these tiny little moments possibly make up for the strain medical school puts on a relationship? They cannot, entirely. You will put up with some absence. But these gestures send the message that our partners are still thinking about us. Maybe they cannot get out of work, but they can say, "I'd rather be with you." They wish they could be at your cousin's wedding, they wish they could be home for dinner, and they wish they could provide you all the affection they would otherwise give. And when they are available, small gestures provide that jolt of appreciation and connection.

Embrace flexibility. Seriously.

When my cousins and I were growing up, my Nana used to take us around town to museums, movies, and restaurants. A recurring theme in our adventures with Nana was the importance of having a Plan B. We never left her house without a backup plan, just in case the movie we wanted was sold out, the store was closed, or the restaurant was packed. Nana's mantra has always been, "You gotta be flexible," a mantra her 12 grandchildren embrace. She is a master of the pivot and when something falls through, she's already moving on to the next adventure. It should not surprise you her husband of 61 years, my Zeide, was an anesthesiologist.

To make the most of your hectic life, you will need to exercise immense flexibility. We need to channel my Nana. We gotta be flexible. Flexibility means pivoting when we need to pivot and adjusting expectations to meet present challenges. Expectations should become *flex*pectations. (See what I did there?!)

If you are a planner, this shift invites pain because it means ceding control to the whims of the medical establishment. But having a backup plan, choosing to have a good attitude, and reframing the situation, can help restore a sense of control. When your partner is suddenly unavailable for outings, reframe your outings as time to spend alone, with friends, or with family. Flexibly changing your attitude and mindset can transform the way you experience an event and minimize the grief caused by your partner's unplanned absence. Decide that you are somebody who has a back-up plan. Then, plan the next time you and your partner will do something together to give yourself something to look forward to. This is not a magical formula to eliminate loneliness and it can take a lot of practice. But it helps.

3. Negotiate constantly

The third ingredient of successful medical couples is consistently renegotiating what time together will look like and what to expect. Successful medical couples must become communication ninjas who constantly communicate and negotiate each person's responsibility for staying in touch, making time for the relationship, and checking in. When one or both of you faces an especially busy stretch, discuss how you are going to keep in touch so that you can keep your relationship strong. Sometimes, relationships enter periods of maintenance. You do not have the time or resources to grow the relationship, so you maintain it while you navigate other areas of life that require your full attention.

When free time becomes scarce, renegotiating might include discussing ways to feel connected despite being apart and saying things like "I miss you. I need more affection when you are in a period of intense studying". Establish that you feel the same way about the issue, and that you both wish you could spend more time together. Frame the conversation in terms of what the two of you can do together to make things better — it is an obstacle for the two of you to face as a team. Nobody is "giving in" or "admitting" to anything because the situation owns the blame.

Building your emotional network

In addition to the work that you will do to maintain open communication and nurture your relationship, build an emotional network to support you when your partner cannot. Here is a list of people whom you can recruit.

Family and friends: Pick people in your life who understand that sometimes you want to vent and sometimes you want advice and do not try to impose on one when you need the other. If you feel frustrated and lonely when your med student cannot come to a wedding or a night out, do not call the family member who will explain to you why your partner cannot be there (you already know) and why you should support them (you already do). This category of support is especially important if you are in a new city.

43

Others like you: I cannot stress this enough — find other people who are dating medical students. It makes a world of difference to have friends who understand your challenges and frustration and can provide emotional support and companionship. Rely on these friends during busy study periods. While conversations will not revolve around your relationships, it may come up and, when it does, these necessary friends will "get it." Once, I invited a friend over for a drink around 6:30 p.m., but she asked if we could reschedule it for 5:00 p.m. sharp. Her partner was on a surgery rotation and he was going to sleep at 8:00 p.m. and she was adjusting her schedule to match his. She walked in, exasperated, and we had an early glass of wine. No problem. As one SO said about other med student partners, "If we want to bitch about [med school], we can. ... If we have to cancel because [my partner] came home early, you understand that." You can enlist your med student to help you find these new friends; they may even feel better about the toll their choices take on you if they have helped you find alternative supports.

Somebody who has been in your shoes: An interesting trend emerged as I interviewed SOs of medical students. Those who knew somebody a few years ahead in medical school and discussed the way medicine impacts a relationship fared much better than those who didn't. Watching somebody go through it can help you gauge your expectations and mentally prepare. On this, one SO said, "We had friends who are in it, two years ahead. It made it easier, you felt more prepared. ... I knew that there would be classes and clinical rotations. I knew that was coming. Seeing that he sometimes had crazy hours, we would not see him, I knew it was going to be crazy." Another SO said that an in-law went through medical school and the family warned them "how difficult it is going to be in terms of how independent you are going to have to be. It was very helpful."

A therapist: Transitions are difficult, and having an unbiased professional to hear you out is extremely helpful. I recommend finding a therapist before you need one. Cultivating a therapeutic relationship takes time, and you will want a strong relationship in place by the time you really need it.

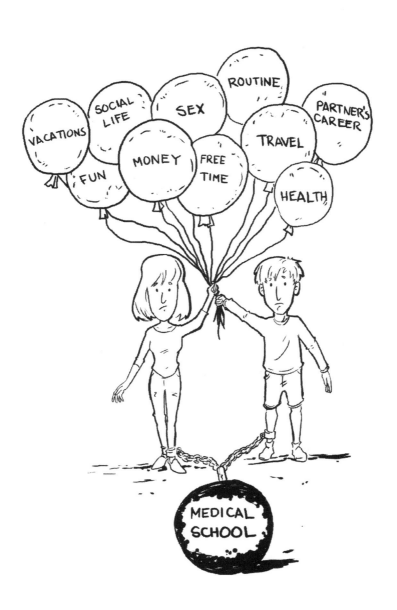

Building this emotional network will help set you up for success in your relationship. We all rely on a large web of support systems to get us through life, and being mindful about stitching this web will make medical school that much easier for you in the long run.

You do you

In addition to building your support system, make sure to have your own life, friends, hobbies, and purpose. If you don't have meaningful things to do when your significant other is totally unavailable, you'll become resentful. Having these things does not mean you will live parallel lives nor is that the goal. Fostering a sense of pride, purpose, and connection can bring the two of you closer together by reaching for happiness both individually and as a unit. Your independence and goal orientation not only benefits you individually but also leads to greater relationship satisfaction. In studies of medical marriages, wives (yes, they haven't done much research on medical husbands) who gave up work outside the home entirely in deference to their husband's profession (or schoolwork) were at much greater risk for dissatisfaction in their marriages. Work outside the home for women married to doctors provides "avenues of social support, stimulation, and individual fulfillment."[17] Not only that, but one of the biggest predictors of happy medical marriages turns out to be mutual support of each other's careers (including homemaking). Medical wives rated their marriages less favorably if they felt dissatisfied with their work/life balance, particularly if they perceived having sacrificed their work or career for family or their husband's career.

In addition to your purpose, it can be helpful to have a list of things you want and need to do when your partner is especially busy. Some examples include:

- Read that book you've been meaning to read
- Hang out with friends that you haven't seen in a while
- Pick up a new hobby or sport

17   Sotile, Wayne M., and Mary O. Sotile. "Physicians' wives evaluate their marriages, their husbands, and life in medicine: Results of the AMA-Alliance Medical Marriage Survey." *Bulletin of the Menninger Clinic* 68, no. 1 (2004): 39-59. doi:10.1521/bumc.68.1.39.27730.

- Start a side business or take on a passion project
- Clean out a closet or room
- Cook a bunch of meals to put in the freezer
- Catch up with people you rarely speak to
- Go out with a group of friends

Flip the script

New goals and projects need not be done in isolation, either. Let your med student in on your new idea, passion, or project so you can discuss it together. Then, fit that passion project into your partner's study time, and let this be a period when you can focus. This makes med school something you use rather than something that uses you. As adults, we lose authority figures who push us to sign up for clubs and activities and try new things. We lose the built-in deadlines of recitals and games to push us to improve at a certain pace. It can be so hard to self-motivate as an adult when there's nobody lighting a fire under your butt. Your partner must spend the next month studying for an exam? Make their exam date your goal date for completing a project. Tell your partner your goal and have them get in on it so when exam day comes, you can both celebrate afterward. Set goals that you want to finish by the time medical school ends. Medical school demands that you bend to its will? Flip the script.

I used this strategy at the beginning of Brian's fourth year of med school. During the summer, he did two rotations at other hospitals around the country, taking him away for two months straight with very limited free time. I decided to start doing insanity workouts, making Brian's return my goal date for completing the 60-day fitness program. I ended up in way better shape when he returned than when he left (just please do not ask me how I'm doing now). That fitness goal was something I wanted to do for myself anyway, but I lacked motivation to start. I used Brian's rotations as a hard deadline. I maximized my alone time and connected with Brian about our shared progress on individual goals. Cheering each other on becomes a great way to build up a relationship.

The advice about preparing plans, and using medical school's structure to your advantage does not imply that you would otherwise be at your partner's beck and call. I know you are not sitting at home reading this, thinking, *Oh! That is what I need! A life! Thank you, Sarah!* Do not mistake this advice as the thoughts of a girl who sits at home eating bonbons and waiting for her husband. (And by the way, what on earth are bonbons and why do people always eat them while they wait?) I followed this advice and developed these strategies while working full-time. I had multiple hobbies and fabulous friends. Flexibility and conscious planning are not signs that you have less going on or have fewer priorities. The men and women I interviewed, the ones who recommended flexibility and patience and struggled with how little they saw their partners, included lawyers, PhDs, doctors, entrepreneurs, salespeople, students, and scientists. Every one of them had full, fulfilling lives that included but were not limited to their partner's endeavors. The fact is, even with full lives, we can still feel the frustrations caused by medical school. We may still feel at the mercy of their schedule.

A brief interlude about housework

One of the biggest time eaters and relationship issue creators is housework. The question of who does how much housework inevitably sprouts from having too little time to do everything you want to do. While this topic may apply more to couples who live together, conflicts over housework can arise with couples who live separately as well. Housework is extremely touchy for many.

Over and over, SOs told me about feeling taken advantage of at home when study periods and rotations got busy. They talked about taking on all household responsibilities, even when they held full-time jobs, went to school full-time, or spent all day caring for children. Almost every SO I spoke with had something to say about housework and the division of labor. Here are some of the comments I received:

- "I work full-time, but he comes home later than I do and he's on his feet all day long and her schedule is more unpredictable than mine.

The second job of the house falls on you. He can be as helpful as he possibly can and still not be that helpful."
- "You are going to feel resentful. Do not turn into their maid."
- "I resented feeling like their maid."
- "I'm home with our new baby and it is crazy. It is really hard. I do everything. I do all the childcare. I do all the shopping, all the laundry, I do everything."

Housework commonly falls to us, causing resentment. One of the hard things is that responsibilities may change over time as the medical student progresses. When your partner has just finished an exam, have them help more around the house and pick up some of the slack. You might say, "So, we've both been really busy lately, but I have been feeling like I do most of the laundry and cleaning. Can we come up with a plan to make sure that we're sharing these responsibilities?" Acknowledge the ebbs and flows of medical school: "When you are on your surgery rotation, do not worry about laundry. We can get back to normal when it ends."

The SOs I spoke to taught me about the importance of finding a non-confrontational way to address housework when it starts to feel unbalanced. Despite our best efforts, we all slide into lazy or inconsiderate behaviors at one point or other. It is so important to be able to bring that up without sparking an argument. One couple I know refers to the sense of shouldering an unfair portion of the household burden as being "dumped on." Whenever one person starts to feel overwhelmed by household responsibilities, they approach the other and say kindly that they are feeling "dumped on." They both know what that means and they can work calmly to solve the problem together.

Other SOs reminded me to reject the idea of an exact 50/50 split of housework. This does not mean that you do all the housework. It means accepting that circumstances may dictate what you and your partner can do during a particular stretch of time. I have fallen into the trap of keeping a mental tally of housework I have done versus what Brian has done (unless, of course, he's done more, in which case, I think, "We should not keep score!"). Obsessing about an even divide will drive you crazy and make you feel resentful or guilty. One SO told me that she knew she and her partner had reached a good place when they were not tallying and they were not keeping score.

I have been through it too! When Brian worked 12-15 hours a day at the hospital during busy rotations, I cooked, cleaned, and did his laundry in addition to working full-time. It wasn't sustainable. I felt resentful and then guilty for my resentment (a quintessential Jewish combination) because I knew he could not help it. Then something happened. I told Brian I was frustrated and he told me he wished he could do more to help. Hearing him say that made me realize how badly I wanted to hear that he saw what I was doing and he appreciated it. Brian began thanking me even more and acknowledging my role in his training. I still did as many loads of laundry, but I felt a lot better about it. Satisfaction is more (not entirely, but more) dependent on perception than concrete equality.

As it turns out, the research supports my feelings. For medical couples, marital satisfaction did not depend on the exact divide of labor in the home or the number of hours the doctor worked. Instead, satisfaction was impacted by spouses' perceptions about how their partners felt about long hours. Basically, spouses felt better about shouldering most the labor if they felt like their spouses understood and felt upset about the imbalance. Even a busy physician (or medical student) can prevent resentment about being unable to meaningfully participate in housework by expressing their frustration with that fact. Here's what the research says:

> Marital satisfaction for physicians' wives were powerfully affected by their perceptions that their husbands made work sacrifices for the sake of their family. Regardless of medical specialty or stage of career, and more than number of hours worked, ... how a busy physician communicates with his wife about the impact of his work on their life appears to have a particularly important effect on his wife's level of marital satisfaction. The finding that, in this cohort of wives who overall gave their marriages positive ratings, 69% stated that their physician husbands regularly expressed distress about their own work/family balance suggests that a physician husband would

be wise to indicate frequently to his wife that he is concerned about the amount of time his work requires him to spend away from their family.[18]

What you decide to do about splitting up housework matters way less than how the two of you discuss it and how you show one another respect. At the heart of my feeling hurt when I carried the load (both figuratively and literally) during long stretches was a sense of loneliness. Gratitude from Brian and his expressed desire to help even when he could not made me feel more like we were in this together. Talking about housework, tackling it together, and renegotiating it when circumstances change, is far more important than who vacuums.

I have a few other thoughts on the subject. During super-busy periods, pinpoint each other's cleaning pet peeves, which can cause disproportionate strain. Maybe you hate seeing dishes in the dishwasher or feel strongly that shoes belong in the closet. During hectic times for both of you, focus on helping one another tackle those pet peeves so, at the very least, you aren't dealing with things that really hit a nerve. Next, find small tasks the busier partner can do to help. They may not be able to vacuum, but they have a few seconds to start the washing machine. Seeing your partner contribute in small ways can help reassure you that they would be helping more under different circumstances. Finally, take on the things that you do not mind doing.

Of course, another solution to the question of housework involves doing less of it. One SO told me that during their first year of marriage, the house absorbed some of the sacrifice. She said, "Sometimes the sacrifice happens to the house, not the relationship. It is better to have a messy house than sacrifice the partner in the relationship. It took time to get acquainted with this concept as newlyweds who had never lived with each other and the added pressure of third-year clinicals."

Sotile, Wayne M., and Mary O. Sotile. "Physicians' wives evaluate their marriages, their husbands, and life in medicine: Results of the AMA-Alliance Medical Marriage Survey." *Bulletin of the Menninger Clinic*, vol. 68, no. 1, 2004, pp. 39–59., doi:10.1521/bumc.68.1.39.27730.

CHAPTER 6
CAN WE TALK?

*"Language, that most human invention, can enable what, in principle, should
not be possible. It can allow all of us, even the congenitally blind, to see
with another person's eyes."*
— *Oliver Sacks*

Communication creates the bedrock of every healthy relationship. Forming
good communication habits and learning how to talk about medical school
and medical subjects can be the difference between gliding and struggling.
Because medical school has shifting schedules and expectations, frequent
check ins are a must. While every relationship requires these conversations,
medical relationships suffer from the reality of more frequent circumstantial
changes. Third- and fourth-year students, for example, begin new rotations
every few weeks or months, each with their own requirements and hours.
Before each transition, check in. These check ins need not be difficult, but
they may include:

How each of you will keep in touch and how often:

Med student: "I will be in the operating room all day so I cannot text you
while I'm in there. But I will do my best to let you know how long I expect to
be there."

Partner: "I'm going to be presenting at a conference this week and I know you
do not have reception at the hospital, so I will call you at the end of the day
to check in."

How you will show affection:

Med Student: "Can we have a hug break every few hours while I study?"

Partner: "I know we will not get to see each other and that you are leaving at 5 a.m., but would you just kiss me goodbye before you leave?"

How you will make time for one another:

Med Student: "I will have 20 minutes tonight before my study group. Can we sit and talk about our days?"

Partner: "OK, you get home at 8 p.m.? I will start scheduling in a snack when I get home from work so we can eat dinner together when you get home."

Who will do what housework:

Med Student: "Can we renegotiate who does what around the house this month? My schedule just changed again."

Partner: "I can manage the laundry until your exam is over."

How you will manage upcoming events:

Med Student: "I do not think I'll be available next Thursday but I'll keep you updated if anything changes"

Partner: "We got invited to a party next weekend, and we have that cousin's wedding next month. Should I RSVP no for you? We were also hoping to have friends over at some point this month. Can you still handle that?"

How you will manage medical-talk at home:

Med Student: "I learned the coolest thing today. Can I tell you about it? Stop me if I get too technical or gross."

Partner: "I know you will be super-stressed about your upcoming test, but can we try not to talk about it all the time? I want to be supportive, but I also want to be able to tell you about what's going on with me."

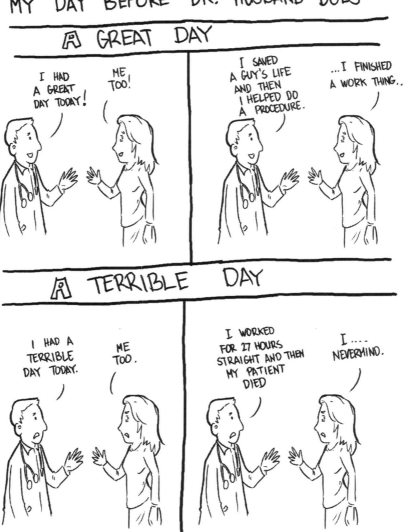

Talking about medical topics

Speaking of which, talk about medicine and medical school will arise, although medical students fall along a spectrum of whether and how much they want to discuss them. Some students get sick of thinking about it and do not want to talk about it when they leave school. One SO (a PhD scientist) told me that she and her partner (a medical student) leave their work at the door and never discuss it at home. Other students rarely stop discussing it — they need to vent about stress, it excites them, or it dominates their thinking.

Med student partners fall on a similar continuum of how much they enjoy hearing about medical school. Some SOs love hearing about classes and learning technical information, while others quickly tire of hearing about the material. One SO said of their past conversations, "I will admit, I tuned him out;...He just rambled. Then I feel bad for not being sympathetic or caring. But sometimes, it is just enough already." Another said, "I do not like drugs and IVs and I do not want to see pictures of surgery. Do not spend 20 minutes telling me exactly what happens to a person's blood pressure." You may love hearing about some aspects of medical school but not others. For example, I enjoyed hearing about the relationships Brian formed with patients and his colleagues, but didn't care to learn about the science. Occasionally, I would tell Brian that I had "reached the limit of my interest" on a topic. Every relationship involves listening to some things you do not find interesting, but with a medical student, that phenomenon can be amplified.

Medical jargon probably will creep into your vocabulary. Medical students learn an endless stream of acronyms and abbreviations to identify different conditions, treatments, and lists of symptoms. On the one hand, learning this jargon may help you feel more a part of your partner's process because it starts to sound less foreign. You may feel more like an insider. On the other hand, you making a huge effort to learn a new language can feel very one-sided. One SO said that to combat the feeling of one-sidedness, they made a deal with their partner. This SO worked in the tech startup world and when medical jargon began dominating the conversation, they said, "You need to know as much about what I do as I know about what you do. You need to know as many tech words as I know medical words."

Gross, graphic stories entail another aspect of medical talk that may enter your relationship. A quick story:

My dad is the oldest of four boys and my grandfather was an anesthesiologist for many years. Apparently, the women who wanted to marry into the family all had to pass the "test" of listening to my grandfather tell gory surgery stories over dinner. My mother tells me about one particular dinner with my grandparents that simultaneously involved hearing a story about intestines coming out of the body and being served spaghetti for dinner.

While my mother passed that test, I assuredly would have failed it. In our home, we have a rule called simply *No Yucky Stuff*. Graphic stories gross me out and occasionally make me feel woozy. We decided that if Brian wants to discuss something graphic, he had classmates who would appreciate hearing his stories. Do not feel bad if you cannot stomach or just do not want to listen to gory stories. That said, unless you set that boundary, the stories will occur and continue. I set this boundary early by saying something like, "I love that you love this stuff, and I love seeing you so excited. But I cannot listen to this. It is too gross for me. I know you may not understand that because it doesn't gross you out, but please respect that I'm asking you not to tell me." Phrasing the request this way accomplished three things:

1) I established my boundaries in a loving way.
2) I told Brian that I wasn't uninterested in him or his line of work. I would just rather eat spaghetti in peace.
3) I preemptively refuted the "I do not get it, it is not that gross" argument because I was asking Brian to adhere out of respect, not out of understanding.

You will need to navigate how much you want to hear about medical school, how much jargon you want to learn, and what kinds of stories you prefer to hear. Like other challenges in medical school, address your partner with kindness and support. Use "I" statements that focus on what you want and do not want to hear, rather than focusing on what they do or do not tell you. That way, they will continue to feel that you care about their journey, even if you can only tolerate hearing about certain aspects of it.

Medical talk in groups of friends

You may start to spend time with your partner's medical school friends. It can be a wonderful experience and make you feel like you are a part of your partner's community. As one SO said, "Being surrounded by community gives me access." Inclusion and connectedness may increase the closeness between you and your partner. I felt this way with Brian's medical school friends. The closer I became to his friends, the more I felt like medical school was ours and not just his. It was also interesting to hear about medical school from his classmates' perspectives so I could get a sense for whether Brian's feelings and experiences were typical.

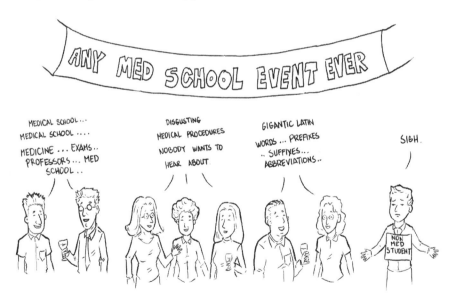

That said, being surrounded by medical students can also lead you to feel isolated, frustrated, bored, and dumb. There were definitely times when I wanted to yell "ENOUGH ALREADY! Can we talk about ANYTHING else, please? Movies, books, politics, religion, farting (no... that would just lead to discussions about farting mechanisms... yes, I have experienced this). If you are already frustrated with the role of medicine and conversations about medicine in your life, being around other medical students may amplify your frustration.

Being around medical students also reopens the conversation about jargon. I noticed, and many SOs mentioned to me how dumb an outsider can feel when sitting with a group of med students. One said, "It is hard being somebody not scientifically minded to get used to being on the outside of the conversation." Another said, "It is sort of a reality to embrace — you are going to feel stupid sometimes. You are going to feel on the outs with the technical stuff." Still another SO recalled a dinner with friends this way: "They are sitting there talking about this doctor, this rotation, this one they had to do an LP on, but the CT was showing this. Like, I have no idea what is happening, and I cannot contribute at all." These conversations isolate all non-medical students and force them to either sit quietly or ask, sometimes over and over, "What does that mean?" "What are you talking about?"

When you encounter medical conversations, try to remember a few things. First, not understanding medical jargon does not indicate a lack of intelligence. If you sat in a room with French speakers and do not speak French, you would be just as confused. You are not dumb if you do not understand what medical students are saying. The only other difference between speaking French and speaking medicine involves the perception we have put on medical students and doctors that what they do is elite, thus elevating their way of speaking to an elite level. Second, remember that everything they say they learned recently, perhaps even yesterday. Medical students do not inherently understand this stuff. If they did, they would probably not have to study for so many hours. They had to learn these things just like anybody else.

You will frequently be put in the position of deciding whether to say something while you sit at a table full of medical students. On the one hand, it is fair to expect a group of people sharing one course of study to discuss it. On the other hand, I believe that those professions with jargon (be it technical jargon, business jargon, legal jargon, or scientific jargon) must be aware of their audience and the fact that some will not understand the words they use. If one person at a table doesn't speak French, it is rude and potentially arrogant for French students to sit around speaking French and exclude that person at the table. It is rude to force people to ask over and over, "what did you say?" "What does that mean?" The same goes for medical students.

The issue of yucky stuff will also arise in social situations involving multiple medical students. I cannot tell you how many times I have stopped a conversation in its tracks because somebody was telling a disgusting story. One SO told me that when they and their partner bumped into a medical school friend, the friend started loudly describing and pantomiming how a C-section looks.

So what can you do if you find yourself frequently addressing incessant medical conversation, too much jargon, and yucky stuff? First, have a conversation with your partner before the next gathering. Explain your feelings of isolation and frustration. As always, make it about how you feel, not what they say. Tell them how much you want to be a part of their social circle and that you would appreciate their help steering the conversation away from technical medical talk and intervening when that does not work. When you are with the group and find the conversation straying too often to unfamiliar, graphic, or technical conversations, ask a question that nudges the conversation in another direction. If subtlety fails, you may have to ask the group, or have your partner ask the group, to change the subject. If a yucky stuff topic comes up that makes you uncomfortable, explain to the group how you feel and turn to your partner for support. Be warned: you may not be taken seriously the first time. They may laugh at you and keep talking. Your next tactic would be to request that they save the story until you are not present or tell the story out of earshot. In the case of yucky stuff, often people genuinely do not realize other people's boundaries. Still others use those stories to sound impressive, to watch you squirm, or to "break you in." If these tactics do not work, you may decide not to spend time with this social group and find other ways to bond with your partner.

Talking about money

I put the topic of personal finance in the communication chapter because many medical couples struggle to have important conversations about finance; in fact, most SOs I spoke to said they either never discussed money or waited to do so when they got engaged. For many, this meant learning about hundreds of thousands of dollars in debt after dating for several years. Now, I'm not advocating that you discuss your debt repayment plan on the first date, but as your relationship progresses, broaching this subject will allow you to make sure you are on the same page and then navigate it together. We don't talk about it, but we know how medical school impacts our finances. Few topics loom larger in a medical student's life and future and I believe both parties should know what they are signing up for.

What does the financial picture look like for the average medical student? According to a 2016 survey by the American Association of Medical Colleges, public institutions cost $36,453 per year and private institutions cost $59,026, before spending for books, rent, food, and other living essentials. Most medical students take out student loans to cover the costs. By graduation, medical students have an average of $189,165 in educational debt, including debt from before medical school. I have spoken with several medical students who casually mentioned having between $250,000 and $300,000 of debt from undergraduate and medical school loans.

Medical students have no monopoly on student debt, but they face an unusual financial trajectory. Many students enter medical school right after college graduation and begin residency in their mid to late twenties. Residencies last between three and seven years depending on the medical specialty and come with a standardized paycheck that starts around $53,500, rising slightly each year. Resident physicians may begin paying back medical school debt, but meanwhile, the interest mounts. After residency, physicians earn an average of $189,000 per year. By this time, many think about buying a home, getting married, or having kids. Some decide to do things while trying to pay off debt. Others attack loans first and postpone other purchases, partially because they get their first real job so late in the game.

Different ways that med students think about loans

Medical students differ in how they think about those loans. Some do not fully comprehend what it means to take out hundreds of thousands of dollars in loans; it is something they must do, and they'll worry about it later. Some obsess about loans, and realizing and resenting the difficult position medical school puts them in, adopt a sort of martyr attitude. One SO described encountering that type of student this way: "Medical school students ... are obsessed with complaining about their loans and obsessed with basically implying that they have it the hardest." Some students treat their student loans like a paycheck or fun money. Brian and I knew people in Miami who spent their loan money on expensive bottle service at South Beach nightclubs. Still others track them meticulously and map out a plan to pay them back as quickly as possible.

The impact of low financial literacy

The current generation illustrates the struggles that come from physicians failing to address finances. According to a 2014 study, over 40 percent of employed doctors worried they would not have enough money to retire, and 45 percent worried they would not be able to fund long-term care expenses. Only 37 percent of doctors considered themselves knowledgeable or very knowledgeable about finance, while 42 percent felt behind on savings goals. About 73 percent of physicians under 40 had student loan debt, and nearly half had $150,000 or more. Of doctors age 40 to 59, 25 percent were still paying back loans. When asked what they would do in hindsight, most physicians would have sought a financial advisor, spent more time on financial planning, and used different investments early in their careers.[19] This does not have to be you and your partner! You can be a good example and start talking, researching, and planning. When you invest in a romantic relationship with a medical student talking about money early on is in your and your partner's best interest.

19 2014 Report on Physicians' Financial Preparedness." 2014 Report on Physicians' Financial Preparedness | AMA Insurance. Accessed May 09, 2017. https://www.amainsure.com/reports/2014-report-on-physicians-financial-preparedness.html.

Medical school does not teach financial literacy, and it defers the natural education that working men and women receive. By the time medical students start residency, and especially when they finish residency, many medical couples are ready to get married (which costs money), have children (which costs money), and buy homes (which costs money). They'll be wrapping their minds around paying off loans and taking out malpractice insurance. Many doctors also run their own businesses, opening private practices or working in partnerships. Some operate sprawling financial enterprises — hiring other staff, managing accounts, and conducting large-scale business. Even doctors who work for large hospitals need to understand how different types of contracts impact their finances. How much money each of you has and how you want to spend or invest it will determine whether you can afford the things and experiences to which you aspire. When Brian and I were dating, we spoke openly about our big-picture finances and discussed how we wanted to use, save, or invest our money. Once we got married we started having monthly budget meetings (Yes, I know what you are thinking: *Wow, Sarah and Brian sound like a very exciting couple.*) and we plan short-term budgets and set long-term financial goals.

Let's make this generation of doctors financially literate and secure. Check out the resources section at the back for tools to help you get started.

A little more about rude comments

As we touched on in Chapter 3, as a med student's partner, conversations about your partner's career will inevitably arise. Strangers, friends, and acquaintances alike will react to your partner's chosen life path. It can be lovely — we get the opportunity to brag about our partners, talk about the struggles we face, and discuss what we're learning about medicine. Unfortunately, you will likely encounter a variety of frustrating and sometimes rude comments. Here are just a few of the actual comments I, my friends, and my interviewees have received when they mention that they are dating/married to a medical student:

- "You will never have to work!" *wink wink*
- "Good catch" *wink wink*

- "Better get a ring on that finger."
- "Do you *ever* see him?"
- "My friend is a doctor, and she has two houses!"
- "Is he in the pocket of big pharma?"
- "Make sure you do everything you can to support his career. Do not interfere."

Yes, these are all insulting in their own special way. Most often, they are not meant rudely, but they almost always come across that way anyway. People sometimes view medical students' SOs as recipients of winning lottery tickets. Well-intentioned acquaintances and friends think it is cute to speak about our imminent financial stability in conspiratorial whispers. Many imply that we date our partners for their financial promise and are excited to rely on their income. Such comments about financial stability stem from the assumption based on doctors' earning potential that your collective life must revolve around medicine. Their comments about you not needing to work betray the assumption that, while the doctor's career choice may be based on fulfillment, ambition, and passion, yours must be based on necessity. Never mind personal ambition, goals, and meaning! I have got a pantry full of bon-bons to eat.

When being asked about your medical student, the next question will inevitably be whether they have picked their specialty, and if so, what it is. (Sometimes they'll assume a decision has already been made and just ask what your partner is going into, even if it is only a month into school.) If your partner has chosen a specialty and you choose to share that information, you are likely to get different reactions based on public perception of the specialty. If it is perceived to be difficult or prestigious (such as neurosurgery), you may get oohs and aahs, some wows, and impressed looks. If you plan to work with children, you may get some "awws," "that is so great," or "that sounds so fulfilling." Every specialty comes with its own reactions and you will soon learn what to expect.

It is not all bad! During our honeymoon, I gushed to strangers about Brian graduating from medical school before our trip began. I could not stop talking about his accomplishment. I looked on admiringly when Brian explained a woman's heart abnormality to her while we took a boat ride in Croatia. He told her why her condition made it harder for her to hike, and she said he'd made her feel better about it now that she understood it better. While buying a souvenir, Brian gave advice to a copper salesman in Sarajevo who asked about a bug bite. I love it. I'm so proud. And that is tough sometimes. Because I'm sometimes the reason medicine gets raised as a topic of conversation and at the end of the conversation, I resent myself for bringing it up.

My attitude about these conversations has run the spectrum. I have fumed with anger at the indignity of being completely overlooked, and I have dwelled with a kindly acquaintance about how amazing Brian's career will be. I noticed that the more comfortable I was with my own career, the easier it became to endure ignorant comments. Still, I sometimes seethe when somebody sends a conspiratorial wink my way.

CHAPTER 7
STANDARDIZED TESTING

"Sometimes, the most brilliant and intelligent minds do not shine in standardized tests because they do not have standardized minds."
— Diane Ravitch

As we discussed, medical school ebbs and flows, and you will encounter stretches of time that involve your partner feeling extreme stress. A few of those times occur prior to taking the medical school standardized tests.

Medical students take a series of standardized tests as they progress throughout their training. You may be familiar with the Medical College Admission Test (MCAT), the standardized test taken before applying to med school. Once in medical school, students start moving through a three-part exam series called the United States Medical Licensing Examination (USMLE), colloquially referred to as "the boards." The individual tests are helpfully named Step 1, Step 2, and Step 3.

In general, medical students take Step 1 at the end of second year, Step 2 at the end of third year or during fourth year, and Step 3 during the first two years of residency. Students are expected to do very well on Step 1 and even better on Step 2. Generally, students study slightly less for Step 2, with the exception being those students who do poorly on Step 1. Students who struggled on Step 1 may need to show tremendous growth in their Step 2 scores to overcome their earlier score.

Osteopathic medical students, going for the DO degree, take their own version of this exam, the Comprehensive Osteopathic Medical Licensing Examination (COMLEX), divided similarly into Level 1, Level 2, and Level 3, which are analogous to the USMLE Step exams and taken at similar points in training. Since most medical students in this country are working toward the MD degree, I will be referring to USMLE and Step exams. But if your partner is a DO student, this chapter applies the same for their exams.

Meet the tests

Step 1 of the boards is eight hours long and tests medical students' understanding of the basic scientific concepts they learned in the classroom through their first two years of medical school. The knowledge tested is both very broad and very detailed and is generally considered to be the hardest test in the series.

For most, studying for Step 1 amounts to the most intensive, stressful studying period of medical school because Step 1 scores carry a lot of weight in residency applications. If your partner already has a specialty in mind, they may look up the average Step 1 score for applicants in that specialty. Typically, the more competitive the specialty, the higher the Step scores required to be competitive in the application process. Better student scores mean more and better options for residency. Because this test is such a big freaking deal, your partner will be under enormous pressure to do well, both for their own future and, if your relationship is serious, your collective future as well.

Step 2 actually consists of two separate tests that may be taken at different times. **Step 2 Clinical Knowledge (CK)** takes the same format as Step 1: it is a nine-hour test taken over the course of a single day. It assesses whether the med student can apply what they've learned on the wards to actual patient care; most questions describe patients and ask questions related to diagnosing or treating them. DO students will take an analogous test, COMLEX Level 2 Cognitive Evaluation.

Both Step 1 and Step 2 CK are multiple-choice exams taken on the computer at an official testing center. There is probably one close to your home, and your partner will probably leave for the testing center in the morning, sit at a computer all day, and return home in the evening. But the other part of Step 2 is entirely different.

Step 2 Clinical Skills (CS) is a practical, hands-on exam lasting about eight hours. Students walk into rooms designed to look like the exam rooms in a doctor's office, where they encounter trained actors portraying sick patients. Students interview and examine them, make diagnoses, and write down what tests or treatments they would order next. The COMLEX equivalent is Level 2 Performance Evaluation. Step 2 CS is a pass/fail exam, and the students who struggle the most are those who do not speak English well.

Because Step 2 CS requires a lot more resources to run than the others, it is only offered in five cities in the whole country: Los Angeles, Houston, Atlanta, Chicago, and Philadelphia (and only the latter two for COMLEX). If you're not lucky enough to go to medical school in one of these cities, taking this test may involve your partner booking a flight and a hotel room, in addition to the over $1,200 cost of the exam itself. (Step 1 and Step 2 CK are themselves over $600 apiece, so everything I've said about discussing finances becomes even more important during exam season.)

Step 3 is another computer-based test, but it won't take place until residency, so you do not have to worry about it for now.

Love in the time of USMLE

In the weeks and months prior to the exam, students may spend many hours each day studying. Though necessary, this study period can be extremely difficult on a relationship. Be prepared to receive very little attention and emotional support during this time. Your partner will be exhausted, frustrated, and overwhelmed. They may become edgy or snappish. As the beginning of that study period draws near (ask your partner when they plan to begin in earnest), you can take some steps both individually and together to prepare.

Talk to your partner about their study schedule: If they have it written out, get a copy of it so you can follow their progress, feel connected to their process, and see what the flow of their plan looks like. Be aware that students may ramp up their study schedules as the test approaches and their strategy may change. As always, flexibility is the name of the game.

Discuss study breaks: Even the most hardcore studiers eat, sleep, and poop. Except for the last one of those, you can use those breaks as your opportunity to spend quality time together. Decide whether you want to try to eat a meal together, have a coffee break, watch TV, or go for a run together. Establishing what makes the most sense for the two of you will make it easier to request their attention when it is time to do those things because you will be on the same page about what you want to do together.

Discuss your "think small" list: Discuss little gestures of affection that you each want while your relationship takes a back seat to studying. You, your partner, and the relationship will still want regular doses of affection to keep you going. It might feel a little weird to talk overtly about needing hugs, kisses, or small touches, but these small gestures make a big difference when you otherwise cannot spend time together. Talk to your partner about what you each love to experience most, and try to incorporate it more frequently.

Shift to thinking about the long term: The health of the relationship will suffer in the short term so that your partner can set themselves up for longer-term success.

Prepare yourself: Now is the time to become busier and mobilize support systems. Plan a project or a goal to tackle during the study time that is unrelated to medical school or your partner. Train for a 5k, paint a picture (or the bedroom), or spend more time with friends. Let friends know that your partner will be unavailable while they study and you will be more available to spend quality time together. Set up weekend activities and get togethers.

Spend time together beforehand: Spend time with your partner before the study binge begins. This will add a little bit of relationship capital into the bank.

If you complete these steps, you will be as ready as you can be to support your studying cave troll. You will have spent quality time together so the two of you will feel fortified and less anxious. You will have plans to stay busy and spend time with others. You will have your partner's study schedule, and the two of you will have discussed breaks and little gestures of affection.

You are likely to provide a lot of one-sided emotional and housework support during this time. In addition to needing moral support, your partner may rely on you to help them cook, do laundry, or make sure they bathe (you think I'm kidding). In high-stress situations like this one, you will want to be aware of the tendency to start comparing stress levels. Watch out for competitive stress. You aren't in a competition with your significant other for who is under the most pressure. You are both stressed out. Some days you will be more stressed out, and some days they will be. Try to be respectful of one another's stress.

CHAPTER 8
THIRD AND FOURTH YEAR

"Happiness does not really depend on objective conditions of either wealth, health or even community. Rather, it depends on the correlation between objective conditions and subjective expectations."
— Yuval Noah Harari

Welcome to the second half of medical school and congratulations on making it this far! Third year and fourth year present the med student with an entirely new paradigm of learning based on clinical experiences. It also presents you and the relationship with new challenges. Third year is viewed almost universally as the toughest year of medical school both for the student and the relationship. Under the tutelage of residents and attending physicians (those who have completed all post-medical school training), students work in different medical specialties, interact with patients in various hospital and office settings, and learn about medicine in a hands-on way. To graduate from medical school, students must complete a certain number of rotation hours, a certain number of required specialties (which differ slightly by institution), and elective hours. At the end of many rotations, students take either a national or school-specific exam.

Third year introduces a slew of new challenges for the two of you to tackle together including frequent schedule and hour changes, even less time spent together, and decreased access to check-ins (hospitals have notoriously bad reception and a wide range of circumstances in which one cannot talk on the phone). We will walk through some of these changes, the implications, and how we can apply our previous messages to these new challenges.

Scheduling the clinical years

Before third year begins, students map out their schedules for the second half of medical school. Here are some of the factors that may go into your partner's decision about how to build their schedule for the next two years.

Specialty: If a student enters third year with an interest in a certain specialty, they will likely take that rotation during third year to try it out and get letters of recommendation before applications, but they may try to avoid taking it at the beginning of third year when they are less experienced, less confident, and less likely to make a positive impression.

Flow: Different rotations have different time, energy, and scheduling demands. Some students structure blocks to avoid grouping difficult rotations together. Others prefer to get tough ones out of the way in a row.

Life events: You may need to schedule rotations around a life event. Brian and I got married during fourth year, so Brian took vacation time around the wedding.

The Match/interview season: During the fall and spring of fourth year, students start attending residency interviews. Most take vacation time to attend these.

Fit: Because different rotations are different lengths, some scheduling ends up being more like a game of Tetris — just find a place where it will fit to make sure it gets done.

The third-year grind

The hours and strain of each rotation vary. While a family medicine rotation may have your partner working a regular 9-to-5, a surgery rotation might require them to work from 5 a.m. to 8 p.m. During each rotation, hours will vary based on the number of patients and what physicians ask them to do. Remember, third-year students are at the bottom of the totem pole and go where they are told. A particularly demanding physician can extend hours by asking the student to do menial tasks. The student really has no choice in the matter. Third-year students frequently work very long hours, put up with bosses who treat the students poorly, and struggle to study for exams. The student's relationship with the physicians they work under also carry higher stakes because those physicians generally assign students' grades and write their letters of recommendation. Students may work overnight or on weekends and holidays, and hours may be unusual or unpredictable.

Third year can batter relationships. Couples see even less of one another, and the two of you cannot settle into a third-year routine because no two rotations are the same. Instead, you and your partner will be adapting and readapting to a new routine every time they switch rotation. Once you acclimate to one weird schedule, your partner starts a new one. On top of all that stress, third- and fourth-year students still go to class, though usually just a few hours a week.

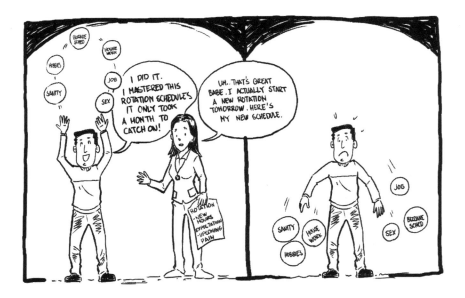

Third year poses the highest risk for burnout. The main factors that cause burnout among third-years include poor clerkship (rotation) organization, cynical residents, and being belittled or mistreated by faculty, staff, and residents.[20]

The systems you've already put in place will help you even more during third year. Make sure you have your alternative supports. Get your partner's schedule, and stay in touch about changes or staying late.

Fourth year

For many, fourth year provides a welcome respite after a difficult year. While fourth-year students continue doing clinical rotations, most students complete the bulk of their difficult rotations during their third year, so their course load lightens up for their final year. Fourth-year students also have the option of doing externships (also called away rotations or audition rotations) to try out other hospitals in their chosen specialty. Choosing a specialty and applying for residency also take place during fourth year.

Externships/away rotations

Fourth-year students may be able to apply to do rotations at other institutions for a few weeks or a month. Externships are tough on a relationship because they force you to navigate long-distance dating, but they are highly strategic in the medical school game. What advantage does doing an externship bring? First, it may clarify to the student what type of hospital setting they wish to practice in. If the medical school is in a suburb, a student may go to a large county hospital to see what the pace and patient population looks like in that setting (in that city). The other reason is that often, programs that accept a student for an externship may be more likely to grant that student an interview for residency, which offers a huge leg up in a competitive process. Ordinarily, programs must judge students based on their written applications and hope that they find students who will resonate with the program. With an externship, not only does the student get to know the people at the institution, but the people working at the hospital get to know the student and

---

20   Dyrbye, Liselotte, and Tait Shanafelt. "A narrative review on burnout experienced by medical students and residents." *Medical Education*, vol. 50, no. 1, 2015, pp. 132–149., doi:10.1111/medu.12927.

determine how they would feel about spending time with them every day.

Brian did two externships:, one in Atlanta and another in Houston. In Atlanta he was invited to interview while he was rotating there during the summer, before he even turned in his residency applications. He came back to Miami with an interview under his belt, which took a little bit of the stress off the process when we started waiting to hear back in the fall. Even though it was stressful having him gone, it was worth it for him to get to explore a few institutions, get a sense for what he liked, and get that early invitation.

Choosing a specialty

By fourth year, medical students are expected to know what specialty of medicine they want to practice and apply to residencies in that specialty. What specialty your partner chooses has a huge impact on their life, your life, and your relationship. When Brian started medical school, I thought people chose a specialty based solely on what they enjoyed learning. Not so. It turns out there are many factors that students consider when they pick a specialty. As you may have a role in the conversation, and even if you do not, understanding how future doctors choose their career path will help you understand their mindset and priorities.

Medicine versus surgery: I did not realize the distinction between medical specialties and surgical specialties. I thought that every type of specialty was "medicine." Well, yes and no. Every specialty is a medical career, but medicine physicians play very different roles than surgeons. Specialties like family medicine, internal medicine, pediatrics, and neurology all fall into the category of "medicine." They generally treat disease with medications and spend their training learning complex thought processes to diagnose and treat illness. Surgeons do some of the things medicine doctors do (you may see an orthopedic surgeon in the office to help figure out why your knee hurts, for example), but their training and practice focus on the technical skill of performing operations and on diagnosing and caring for patients who have had surgery or will need it soon. Although some specialties involve a combination of medicine and surgery and others fall outside of this binary, most students must decide which of these two focuses appeals to them more strongly.

Interest: What topics does your partner get really excited about? Do they love studying the brain? The kidneys? One of the scary things about choosing a specialty is that, with a few exceptions, doctors generally stay put with their specialty so it is vital to pick something they enjoy.

Adults versus children: Some prefer to work with children (and parents!) while others prefer working with adults.

Relationships to patients: Different types of doctors have different types of relationships with patients. A primary care physician gets to know their patients over the course of many years. A specialist interacts with patients on a specific basis, with a mix of short-term and long-term patient relationships. Anesthesiologists rarely get to know patients well; they do most of their work while the patient is asleep or sedated. Emergency physicians see lots of different patients but do not form any long-term bonds. Most radiologists never see patients; they sit in a room and read x-rays all day. One crucial factor in choosing a specialty is deciding what type of relationship they want with patients and how vital that component is to their job satisfaction.

Money: Different specialties come with different pay scales. They are all relatively high, but still range widely.

Lifestyle and flexibility: Different specialties result in different lifestyles. Some are 9 a.m. to 5 p.m.; others require longer hours. Many specialties require being on call at certain times, meaning the physician must stop what they are doing and go to the hospital when they are called. Some specialties work longer hours than others, and some have longer training periods. A person should consider lifestyle when they pick a specialty. It is also important to look at the training demands versus demands after residency. Some specialties require many years of training but offer excellent hours once residents graduate. Some specialties afford more flexibility around vacation time, hours of operation, and appointment times.

Competitiveness: Some specialties are more competitive. To get into very competitive specialties, a medical student needs excellent grades, outstanding Step 1 and 2 scores, recommendations, and sometimes additional years of research.

Personality type: Different personality types are (sometimes) attracted to different specialties. Of course, there are no hard rules, but there are medical stereotypes about what personality chooses what specialty. When your partner starts doing rotations, they'll see what kind of people they interact with during each rotation. They may find they are drawn to a specialty based partially on which doctors and residents they connect with best. Medical students choose their colleagues when they pick a field.

Gender: Gender has been shown to impact specialty choice. Historically, female medical students have been more motivated by direct patient contact and pursue specialties that offer more flexibility and the ability to work part-time, which may explain why women tend to be under-represented in surgery and overrepresented in primary care, pediatrics, psychiatry, and obstetrics and gynecology. Men, in contrast, are more often motivated by technical skills or career opportunities."[21] Another study found that both male and female medical students expected that the woman's career would be impacted by parenthood, but that the men would be unaffected.[22]

---

21   Alers, Margret, Petra Verdonk, Hans Bor, et al. "Gendered career considerations consolidate from the start of medical education." *International Journal of Medical Education* 5 (2014): 178-84. doi:10.5116/ijme.5403.2b71.
22   Buddeberg-Fischer, Barbara, Martina Stamm, Claus Buddeberg, et al. "The impact of gender and parenthood on physicians' careers - professional and personal situation seven years after graduation." *BMC Health Services Research 10*, no. 1 (2010). doi:10.1186/1472-6963-10-40.

CHAPTER 9
THE MATCH

"Human knowledge is never contained in one person. It grows from the relationships
we create between each other and the world, and still it is never complete."
— *Paul Kalanithi, When Breath Becomes Air*

Your partner has chosen a specialty and is ready to start the application process? Woo. Grab a beer and I will explain how this all works. Got your beer? No? Go get one.

Medical students submit applications to residencies through a process called The Match, which for most specialties is run by the National Resident Matching Program. Once again, the specifics differ slightly for students in osteopathic programs, as well as students in the military and those applying to certain specialties that run their own match, but the overall process is the same. Here's the basic layout:

In the fall of their fourth year of medical school, students apply to residency training programs in their chosen specialty. Residencies read the applications and choose students to interview for their limited number of residency spots. Students receive email interview invitations and go on interviews between October and February. After interview season ends, students and programs each compile rank-ordered lists. Students rank programs from most to least preferable through an online portal. Programs do the same, ranking students from most to least preferable. An algorithm matches students and programs based on these preference lists, slightly favoring the students' desires over the residencies'.

It is all very confusing and I highly recommend you read more about it. I've left links to in-depth explanations in the resources section. On a specified

Monday in mid-March, students receive an email telling them whether they matched. That Friday, students who match find out where they will be assigned. Students are contractually obligated to go to the residency where they match. Some students always fail to match, though the percentage is small. If your partner doesn't match, they enter a process called the Supplemental Offer and Acceptance Program, or SOAP. When a student SOAPs, they enter a free-market system where they go through a quick succession of interviews with programs that have empty spots left. Over the course of the four days between when students are informed about whether they match and that Friday, Match Day, SOAP students accept or decline offers from programs with open spots. Students who fail to SOAP may take a year off for research or work and reapply to the Match the following year.

Why do residency applications work like this?

From the outside, the match system does not seem to make any sense. Why do applications work this way? Why can't students apply to residencies the way they apply to other jobs? Here's why:

The National Resident Matching Program started in 1952 in response to pervasive application issues when residency applications functioned in a decentralized, competitive market. In a free-market system, hospitals started scouting and recruiting top first- and second-year medical students (kind of like college sports). Students were asked to commit to programs years before they could apply. Hospitals benefitted by filling residency spots early, but students who received these offers lost the opportunity to look at competing offers. In 1945, medical schools delayed releasing transcripts and recommendations to prevent hospitals from early scouting. Hospitals responded by offering spots to students later but demanded that students commit within 12 hours of receiving an offer; some even demanded a decision while the student was still on the phone. The Match was created in 1951 to address the system and give hospitals and students the opportunity to see their options and rank their preferences.[23]

---

23 Gusfield, Dan, and Robert W. Irving. "The stable marriage problem: Structure and algorithms." Cambridge Mass.: MIT Press, 2003.

Process costs

Residency applications, much like everything else in medical school, come with a shocking price tag. Medical students invest many hours considering dozens of potential program options, and then pay for each application. Once programs are chosen, there is a centralized application process, reducing the time intensiveness of that step of the process. To combat the ease of applying to dozens of programs, each application comes with a cost per application that rises the more applications a student sends.

The number of programs a student applies to will vary from person to person depending on the quality of their application (based on Step scores, grades, recommendations, etc.), the competitiveness of the specialty, and how secure or insecure the applicant feels about their chances (if a student feels insecure or uncompetitive, they may apply to more programs), and application costs. Given that many students apply to 30-50 programs, depending on the specialty and the competitiveness of the student's application, the price of initial applications will be hundreds of dollars.

In addition to the initial interview costs, the system encourages students to go on a lot of interviews to give themselves the highest possible chance of matching. Students usually have to foot the bill for transportation to and from the interviews, accommodations in those cities, and associated travel expenses. By the end, many invest thousands of dollars into the residency application process.

Interview season

Residency applications open on a specific day in September, and students work to have all the components of their application ready to send on that first day. Students may start to hear back from programs in early or late fall and from there, they begin planning their interview season. Many residencies use a tiered interview invitation system that sends out a batch of interview invitations to the program's top-pick students, who then have the opportunity to schedule their interview slots. When interview slots open up due to cancellations or declined invitations, they send out a batch of invitations to the next tier of students on the list. This means students can receive new interview invitations in the middle or at the end of interview season. Last-minute interviews can cost more (less notice) and have less flexibility of interview dates.

Making the rank list

After interview season concludes, you and the applicant may find yourselves sitting and discussing the rank list for residency. How you rank the programs will depend on your priorities. Here are some of the factors to consider:

Location: Where do you and your partner want to live? Where do you want to work? Are you applying to schools or jobs? Where do you have easiest access to family and friends and a support system? These as well as cost of living and weather will differ depending on your location.

Program prestige: Prestigious programs can open doors later. Those who want to work in academic hospitals may also pay closer attention to program prestige.

Teaching style/philosophy: Every program has a vibe.

Curriculum: Residency programs are standardized in what they must teach, but there is wiggle room, and each program has a slight variation on the theme. A curriculum loaded up with a particular type of rotation or with lots of built-in research time may strongly attract one applicant and drive away another.

Program size: Some want larger programs with more colleagues and possibly more amenities. Others prefer a smaller environment.

Hospital type: A county hospital in the middle of a city brings in different patients than suburban hospitals.

The relationship stress of match interview season

Going through the match season creates relationship stress in several different ways. Logistically, the process punctuates the school year with the additional responsibility of applications, interviews, rank list creation, and Match week. Students often use days off to attend interviews, giving them even less free time than usual. The financial stress is no small consideration. Also, once again, medicine forces you to get on the same page about the stage of your relationship. Where your relationship stands may determine what role you have in their application process and how the two of you think about each of your trajectories. For new couples and deeply committed couples, the conversation may not be relevant at all, or have taken place months prior to the process beginning. In between lies a wide range of relationships with no determination of long-term trajectory.

Dealing with the questions surrounding your relationship while your partner begins a deeply vulnerable application process that puts all their hard work on the line can be difficult. If possible, discuss these questions before the student starts to send in their initial application. Much like the application process for medical school, even couples who do every step of the application process together will find that this process looks different. Sit down together and list out your priorities.

If the two of you make a rank list together, you will have to incorporate many of the factors listed above. A couple may have to weigh competing priorities such as a job opportunity for you in one city versus a more preferable residency in a different city. Or you may agree to sacrifice that job opportunity so that your partner can pursue their dream program. Setting out your priorities together can lead to quite a bit of stress.

You will also be dealing with the stressful reality that if you intend to live in the same city as your partner, a computer algorithm will ultimately decide where you end up next. If you are applying to graduate school, you and your partner may have to coordinate where you apply. If you work, you will either job hunt in multiple cities or wait until Match Day to start the hunt in the confirmed city.

I spoke with SOs who were going through different versions of this stress. Some I spoke with were in the middle of graduate school, unable to leave if their partner got assigned elsewhere. Others were eager to leave and start over someplace new or closer to home. One SO reflected on the implications of the Match to their job this way: "The most challenging part is that your career is dependent on where we match. Wherever we go, I must figure it out also. ... It is the most challenging part. ... Your aspirations have to come second." While Brian applied to residency, I applied to graduate school so we coordinated our processes and frequently discussed our priorities. Fortunately, he prioritized my career goals in addition to his own. But even still, the reality remained that, assuming Brian matched, he would be guaranteed to move along to the next step of his career, while I might or might not get into graduate school in the corresponding city.

SOs told me about different approaches and levels of involvement that they had with the match process. Thinking his girlfriend would end up in a particular city, one SO got a job in that city to prepare for his girlfriend's predicted arrival. A married SO described being almost entirely left out of the process, her husband ranking programs and consulting her at the end, even though his top choice moved her to a new city, farther from family, with small children, while she finished graduate school. A third said she wanted to stay where they were, where she had built a thriving career, but her spouse didn't receive interviews locally. A fourth couple decided that the student should apply all over the country, even though the student's partner needed to stay put to complete a PhD. There are so many possible scenarios. All you can do is be honest with one another about your priorities and make the best possible list for the two of you.

Waiting: The worst part of the process comes in the time between sending in a rank list and waiting for Match Day, about a month. On the one hand, the outcome is no longer in your control. On the other hand, the outcome is no longer in your control! You may find that the two of you are thinking constantly about the possibilities. Some people excel at training their minds not to think about an impending event. I envy those people. The best you can do is to stay busy and employ the same systems you use when you want to avoid feeling like you are waiting for your partner to finish studying. Take on a project, spend more time with friends, rely on support systems, and reframe the situation to think about the relief of finishing that process.

Match Day: On the Friday of Match Day, schools receive all the envelopes stating where their students will train and are allowed to give them out to the students starting at noon Eastern Time. Then, at 1 p.m., an email goes out to the applicants telling them where they got in. Most schools have Match Day ceremonies and traditions that involve students learning their future in a room with others and possibly even on stage, one at a time. For the school, these traditions foster pride in the accomplishments of their students and foment communal celebration. For students who match at a top choice, it can be a wonderful thing to learn of your destination surrounded by friends and sometimes, family members who attend the ceremony.

For all the good intentions, however, these traditions overlook the struggle that a student might encounter as they discover they matched at their last-choice program in front of a crowd of happy classmates. Matching culminates all of a medical student's hard work and often represents a huge life step for individuals and couples who go to new cities and institutions. Ceremonies turn an intensely private moment into a public spectacle. Be aware of this fact, because you or your partner may be forced to process an intense emotional reaction, be it joy or sadness, in front of others. That is not an easy thing to do.

When Brian matched, he and I walked on stage in front of a giant tent full of people, including his family, who flew in for the occasion. It was a lot to take in, and I got overwhelmed. After we learned onstage that he matched at a top choice, I found myself needing to process the experience in a more intimate setting. I found a close friend who attended the ceremony and asked her to go get coffee with me. That evening, I expected to want to party, but I needed quiet. Months of thinking about possible destinations, new homes, where we would be in relation to family, how this would impact my career and graduate school choices, all came together in an exhausting rush. We had our answer, and it was a great one. But the weight of the previous months hit me that day and I needed time alone and time with Brian. It is ok if you also feel overwhelmed. It is a lot.

CHAPTER 10
CONCLUSIONS AND NON-CONCLUSIONS

*"We don't become better because we acquire new information. We become better
because we acquire better loves. We don't become what we know. Education is a process
of love formation. When you go to a school, it should offer you new things to love."*
— David Brooks, The Road to Character

There is so much I have not said. There is more research to conduct, more
dynamics to explore, and more interviews to be done. I can name dozens of
topics I did not cover but could have included in this book — having children, dynamics between significant others and families, race and ethnicity in
medical school, international medical schools, military med students, transitioning into residency, healthcare policy… the list goes on and on. I could
either be daunted by the task or grateful for the opportunity to continue writing. This guide is neither perfect nor complete, but it is something.

Wittingly or unwittingly, we are entwined in the American medical subculture. We are spectators and participants.

In closing, I'd like to share my Facebook post from the day before Brian
graduated from medical school:

> Tomorrow, Brian graduates from medical school and officially
> becomes a doctor! These last four years have not been easy.
> Medical school is brutal for students and tough for those who love
> them. Students endure hours and hours of studying and rotations,
> necessitating single-minded focus on academic and clinical success.
> Medical school demands all a student's time, energy, and money.
> There are times when students are lucky to get 6 hours of sleep and a

shower. It has sometimes felt unnecessarily brutal — a hazing ritual by the gatekeepers who themselves were hazed by their superiors. As your girlfriend, fiancée, and now wife, I have done my best to support you through it all.

Dating/marrying a medical student can be confusing, frustrating, and lonely. We are unbelievably proud of your achievements while resenting the system that makes you physically and emotionally unavailable. We fall in love with your drive and passion even as our relationships can become a casualty to your ambition. We love people's admiring reactions to your status and endure well-meaning but insulting comments to hold on to you because you are our ticket to financial stability. We love learning from you, and we sometimes space out when you get too detailed or graphic. We are independent men and women with our own goals and individual lives and interests who are experts at building alternative support systems, taking on new projects, and building thriving careers in cities we must live in so you can finish school. We work constantly to reconcile our own ambitions with the fact that medicine must often be prioritized. We are expert planners, preparing hobbies and outings for those weeks when you will be working overnight shifts… again. But we love you.

And Brian, I love you so much it overwhelms me. I have watched you learn, and I have learned so much from you. I have watched you grow in confidence and have been (mostly) happy to be your human pin cushion to help you practice. It makes my heart burst when I see how happy and fulfilled your work in medicine makes you. Tomorrow is your accomplishment and our triumph, and I cannot wait for what's next for you and for us. Mazal tov, my Brian.

RESOURCES

Med Student burnout resources:
studenthealth.emory.edu/hp/documents/pdfs/distress_resources.pdf
thehappymd.com/blog
pamelawible.com/

Medical partner online resources:
reddit.com/r/MedSpouse/
physicianfamilymedia.org
nurturingmedicalmarriage.com
doctorswives.org/
kevinmd.com
livesofdoctorswives.org

Financial Resources tailored to med student and physician needs:
whitecoatinvestor.com
drwisemoney.com
MDMag.com
WealthyDoc.com
SmartMoneyMD.ocm

Other medical relationship books
The Medical Marriage: A couple's Survival Guide- Wayne Sotile & Mary Sotile
Medical Marriages- Glen Gabbard M.D. & Roy Menninger M.D.
At Least You will be Married to a Doctor- Jordyn Paradis Hagar, MSW
Doctors' Marriages: A Look at the Problems and Their Solutions- Michael Myers
Surviving Residency: A Spouse's Guide to Embracing the Training Years, Kerstin Math
The White Coat Investor: A Doctor's Guide to Personal Finance and Investing – John Dahle, M.D.

General Relationship Books:
The Seven Principles for Making Marriage Work- John Gottman, Ph.D
Hold Me Tight- Dr. Sue Johnson
The 5 Love Languages: The Secret to Love that Lasts- Gary Chapman

ACKNOWLEDGEMENTS

When taking on a big, unfamiliar project, my greatest obstacle is Imposter Syndrome — that voice telling me that I am not qualified, talented, competent, or persistent enough to do what I am doing. Countering that voice can feel like a full-time job. Fortunately, I surround myself with the most wonderful people who remind me of my worth and my voice.

The single most important person I need to thank is my husband, Dr. Brian Fromm. He steadfastly supported me throughout this project and talked me through my fears. He spent hours editing drafts and correcting the small details I tend to miss. He held my hand through my insecurities. Imposter Syndrome is no match for a loving husband.

I would also like to thank my family and friends who supported me throughout the writing process. Sarah Goliger, Rachel Weinstein, and Gabbi Lewin have been my cheerleaders and advisors. I could not have finished this book without their ongoing support. My immediate family — Mom, Dad, Benjamin, and Sam, have become familiar with my ceaseless search for new challenges. Their faith in me makes striving feel less cary. I want to thank my fantastic in-laws Susan Fromm, Alan Fromm, Julie Abergel, and Josh Abergel. I could not have married into a more loving or supportive family.

I feel grateful to have found such a wonderful editor, Douglas Williams, who shook my writing out of its rut, and pinpointed my issues with tone, flow, and wording. He provided me with fresh perspective, helped me weave together a story, and cleaned up the writing. He was professional and prompt and I'm incredibly grateful. I want to thank my cover designer Andy Highland, for creating a dynamic book design that avoided being cliché, predictable, or girly. Glass84, even though I don't know your name, I'm grateful to you for bringing my cartoons to life.

I would also like to thank the men and women who let me interview them for this book. You let me into your life and your relationships with openness and vulnerability. You shared your deepest struggles, anxieties, and fears and I learned something new from every single interview. The insights you gave me are peppered throughout this book. For confidentiality reasons, I will not list your names, but please know that this book would not have been nearly as insightful without your input.

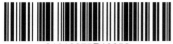

Made in the USA
San Bernardino, CA
10 July 2018